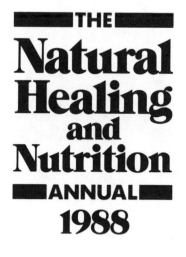

THE
Natural
Healing
and
Nutrition
ANNUAL
1988

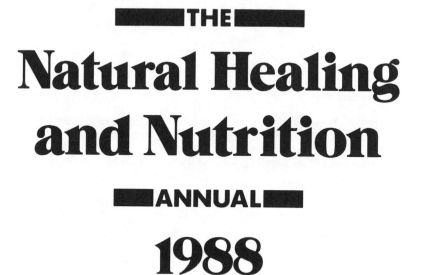

THE

Natural Healing and Nutrition

ANNUAL

1988

Edited by MARK BRICKLIN,
Executive Editor, *Prevention*® Magazine

Written by the Staff of Rodale Press

Rodale Press, Emmaus, Pennsylvania

Printed in the United States of America on recycled paper
containing a high percentage of de-inked fiber.

ISBN 0-87857-743-2   hardcover

2 4 6 8 10 9 7 5 3 1   hardcover

Contents

Nutrition and Health Bulletins

The Healing Power of Nutrition

Niacin: A Happy Surprise for the Heart
Used in drug-strength doses, this vitamin can clean up
blood fats and lengthen life.   130

The Health Power of Perfect Sleep
Specialists have new answers to an old problem—
answers that can make you feel better and perform
better all day.   135

Stroke-Prevention Surgery: How Safe Is It?
Doctors now suspect that for many patients, the
risks of this popular operation may outweigh the
benefits.   142

Weight-Loss and Fitness Updates

Walk Off Your Hips and Wake Up Your Health!
Scientists have found the positive effects of this most
natural of all sports to be awesome. It helps everything
from bad circulation and a bum back to a plain old
pot belly!   147

Lose a Little, a Little More, a Little More . . .
The take-it-easy philosophy often works better than
declaring WWIII against your bulges.   153

How to Get the Most "Slimming Power" from the Rotation Diet
Even the best diet may ultimately fail, say our experts,
unless a few "special ingredients" are in your plan. . . .   157

Make Weight Loss Easier with Some Spouse Psychology
Is your partner in life a hindrance in slenderizing?
Shape up his (or her) attitude and watch your own
shape improve.   164

Looking Good

The Practical Psychology of Positive Living

SUPPLEMENTS AND COMMON SENSE

Some of the reports in this book give accounts of the professional use of nutritional supplements. While food supplements are in general quite safe, some can be harmful if taken in very large amounts. Be especially careful not to take more than these commonsense limits:

Vitamin A	20,000 I.U.
Vitamin B_6	50 mg.
Vitamin D	400 I.U.
Selenium	100 mcg.

NOTICE

The information and ideas in this book are meant to supplement the care and guidance of your physician, not to replace it. The editor cautions you not to attempt diagnosis or embark upon self-treatment of serious illness without competent professional assistance. An increasing number of physicians are ready to cooperate with clients who want to improve their diet and lifestyle; if you are under professional care or taking medication, we suggest discussing this possibility with your doctor.

Introduction:
Keeping Healthy
in the Age of Confusion

You might think that in today's world, the challenge of caring for your health would be a lot simpler than it was a thousand years ago.

But only if you didn't really think about it.

Consider for a minute all the theories that are advanced and debated about nutrition and health: All the controversy over vitamin supplements . . . confusion about exercise regimens . . . the mind-numbing array of over-the-counter medications at your local drugstore . . . the near-miraculous, half-tested, have-they-recalled-it-yet assortment of powerful new pharmacologicals.

We're better off, for sure, than even the mightiest kings of the Middle Ages, when it comes to health. But in a way, we're even more confused. The Age of Certainty in medical care never really came. Instead, we live in the Age of Options. Options that are in our own hands, our own minds.

This book is devoted to helping you exercise those options with knowledge and common sense. Some call it self-care. Some call it personal empowerment. The idea is that health is not something that is handed to you but something you make for yourself.

Do you know how to make yourself a good dinner? Sure. To a point. But do you know about the option that says: your dinner can have an important effect on how you feel tomorrow? On how long you will live in good health? Do you know about the specific foods that can have a strong effect on cancer, on your blood vessels, on your ability to think, even on arthritis?

That information is here, all in one place. Suddenly, some of the confusion begins to clear up.

Like many people, you're probably interested in vitamins

and healing herbs. But do you know how much is enough, and when you're on the brink of danger? Do you know the herb that can help prevent blood clots? The mineral deficiency that can cause headaches and brittle nails? The vitamins that help inflamed gums? The vitamin that teams up with a certain food fiber to pull down blood cholesterol?

That information is here, too. And a little more confusion evaporates.

Remedies from the environment don't stop at those sold in food markets. There are drugstores, too. Faced with a maddening allergy, you may also be faced with a maddening number of options. Do you know when you really need an antihistamine? Is a prescription drug truly better than the over-the-counter variety? And should you be taking an antihistamine or a decongestant? Or both? Do you know the special danger of decongestants to older men? Do you know which cold medications make you sleepy and which counteract sleepiness?

All that information is here, too. The confusion is gone. And hopefully, so is that runny nose!

Please enjoy your 1988 *Natural Healing and Nutrition Annual.*

Mark Bricklin
Executive Editor
Prevention® Magazine

Nutrition and Health Bulletins

HEALTHIER ARTERIES WITH FISH OILS

For the first time, scientists have found that fish oil can slow the formation of arterial deposits, which are the primary cause of heart attacks and strokes.

Researchers at the University of Chicago fed a diet high in fish oil to 16 rhesus monkeys, who developed far fewer arterial deposits (plaque) than 8 monkeys fed a diet high in coconut oil, a saturated fat known to contribute to the development of atherosclerosis.

The plaque that did develop in the monkeys that were fed fish oil was found to be less likely to cause medical complications and contained fewer inflammatory cells, according to the researchers. Levels of LDL (low-density lipoprotein) cholesterol—considered a risk factor for heart disease—were also lower with the fish-oil diet.

Other studies have found that fish oil can lower blood cholesterol and inhibit blood clotting. This study marks the first time that researchers actually measured the effects of fish oil on the arterial wall, according to Robert Wissler, M.D., Ph.D., professor of pathology at the University of Chicago.

The researchers, who don't know why fish oil has this beneficial effect on arterial walls, recommend that people replace the saturated fat in their diet at least once a day with a marine oil source. Dr. Wissler says he does this himself, substituting cold-water fish, such as sardines, tuna and salmon, for meat.

VITAMIN E
FIGHTS TUMORS

Harvard University researchers, in a recent study, found that vitamin E can prevent tumors in hamsters that are exposed to small amounts of a potent carcinogen.

The vitamin, when given to the animals exposed to larger amounts of the cancer-causing substance, inhibited but did not prevent tumor growth.

The scientists divided the hamsters into four groups. The first two groups were exposed to small amounts of the carcinogen, the third was given only vitamin E and the fourth group, which was given nothing, was used as a control. Of the first two groups, group one received ten milligrams of vitamin E every other day. In between, the hamsters were exposed to the carcinogenic chemical. Group two was exposed to the same amount of the chemical but was not given the vitamin E.

After 22 weeks, the second group all had tumors of varying sizes, but group one had no tumors at all *(Journal of Dental Research)*.

VITAMIN C MAY HAVE SPECIAL BENEFITS FOR DIABETICS

Everybody's skin needs collagen to build on. Collagen, a protein, gives skin — along with bones, gums and other tissues — its strength.

For most of us, collagen comes naturally. But diabetics have trouble producing this essential protein. As a result, they don't heal as quickly as people without diabetes. Their skin also grows older faster, and they have more gum disease.

But if you're diabetic, recent research at the University of Southern California (USC) may someday save your skin. Scientists at the university have found that diabetic mice, fed large doses of vitamin C, produce more and higher-quality collagen.

Why? Vitamin C simply makes collagen much more stable. But in diabetics, not enough vitamin C makes its way into the body's cells. That's because sugar, which rises to abnormally high levels in diabetics, competes with vitamin C for entry into the cells. The higher the blood sugar rises, the less vitamin C enters the cells.

"The relationship between vitamin C and sugar has been well documented," says Michael Schneir, Ph.D., head of biochemistry at the USC School of Dentistry, who led the study. "One of the results, slow healing, is a major problem with diabetics."

This study does not suggest diabetics begin taking large doses of vitamin C. Studies in people have yet to duplicate the USC findings in rats. Other studies, however, have demonstrated an important link between vitamin C and collagen-related disorders such as gingivitis, according to Dr. Schneir. "These things are all starting to add up," he says.

LOW MAGNESIUM
LINKED TO SUICIDE

Could a magnesium deficiency make you suicidal?

Suicidal patients studied by a group of Hungarian scientists had lower-than-normal levels of magnesium and a substance that indicates the presence of a calming brain chemical in their cerebrospinal fluid.

What's significant about this finding is that it is the first time researchers have linked low levels of the mineral magnesium — believed necessary for the production of the brain chemical serotonin — to low levels of the substance 5-hydroxyindoleacetic acid (5-HIAA), which is a by-product of serotonin production.

According to previous research studies, low levels of 5-HIAA may possibly be an identifying marker for suicide. In any case, it is an indication of low serotonin levels, which tend to be common in patients who have previously attempted suicide.

The researchers suspect further investigation may show that magnesium plays a role in some mental disorders and, possibly, in suicidal behavior, as it relates to the body's production of serotonin *(Biological Psychiatry)*.

FISH FIGHTS
BLOOD FATS

Adding fish to your diet may reduce the amount of cholesterol in your blood, even if you eat more cholesterol-rich foods than you should.

That's the finding of an Australian researcher who fed six healthy volunteers almost three egg yolks daily, along with about 2½ tablespoons of fish oil. Despite the addition of egg yolk to the diet, the blood cholesterol levels of the volunteers remained at healthy levels.

Fish oils are rich in highly unsaturated omega-3 fatty acids, which appear to prevent blood platelets from sticking together and forming dangerous clots. These clots can lodge in an artery and cause a stroke or heart attack.

But in this study and in a number of previous reports, omega-3 acids also seemed to block the body's production of LDL (low-density lipoprotein) cholesterol. Tiny globs of LDL predispose the arterial walls to the formation of plaque. Over time, plaque buildup blocks blood flow and decreases the amount of oxygen getting to the brain and heart

One of the most intriguing results of this study was a dramatic lowering of plasma triglycerides, artery-clogging blood fats. Polyunsaturated vegetable fats also lower triglycerides, but the drop triggered by omega-3 fatty acids is "far greater," says researcher Paul J. Nestel, M.D., of the Baker Medical Research Institute *(American Journal of Clinical Nutrition)*.

COFFEE CREAMERS CAN CLOUD YOUR BLOOD

If you're trying to cut down your cholesterol intake by whitening your coffee with a cholesterol-free nondairy creamer, hold your spoon for just a minute.

Researchers at the University of Nebraska Medical Center point out that, while nondairy creamers are technically "cholesterol free," they contain other substances that, in combination, cause a "marked and persistent" elevation in blood cholesterol in laboratory animals.

In particular, coconut oil, found in many creamers, contains a higher proportion of cholesterol-raising saturated fat than butter.

The researchers estimate that if you add a teaspoon of nondairy creamer to the ten cups of coffee you consume a day—itself a bad idea—you add 100 calories of "hidden" and very saturated fat.

This is especially important news for Americans, who drink 33 million gallons of coffee each day—equivalent, the researchers note, to 30 seconds of full flow of Niagara Falls *(New England Journal of Medicine).*

WITH E,
THEY CAN SEE

Children born with the disease abetalipoproteinemia can't absorb fat efficiently. As a result, they have trouble absorbing fat-soluble vitamin E unless it is given in very large doses. Left untreated, this vitamin E deficiency can lead to blindness.

The retina—the light-gathering area of the eye—contains polyunsaturated fatty acids. The interaction of light and oxygen with these fatty acids creates microscopic cell killers called free radicals. These free radicals wreak havoc with the cells of the retina. In the eye, vitamin E neutralizes free radicals and prevents them from damaging cell membranes, the cell's skin.

Armed with this knowledge, doctors at the Hospital for Sick Children in London enlisted daily supplements of vitamin E in their efforts to save the sight of six patients. These patients were studied over long periods, in one case up to 18 years. In each case, doctors were able to keep the patients from losing their sight.

SHORT ZINC, SMALL BABIES

If you're a mother-to-be, getting enough zinc in your diet could mean the difference between a normal, healthy baby and one that is abnormally small.

According to researchers at St. Thomas Hospital in London, zinc deficiency in pregnant women might be linked to intrauterine growth retardation in their babies.

Zinc affects the production of natural fatty acids in the body called prostaglandins. These body chemicals are necessary for fetal growth.

Doctors suspect that in the women they studied, zinc deficiency hindered production of prostaglandins in the placenta and prostacyclin, a potent vasodilator, in the umbilical cord.

The 17 mothers under study, all of whom gave birth to very small infants, had significantly lower concentrations of zinc than mothers who had normal babies, according to the report *(Pediatric Research)*.

ARTHRITIC BRUISING?
CHECK VITAMIN C

Spontaneous bruising is usually considered an unfortunate but inevitable side effect of rheumatoid arthritis, a crippling joint disease that tends to leave the skin fragile. But two British rheumatologists suggest that instead of accepting skin hemorrhaging as part of the disease, physicians should look for another cause: vitamin C deficiency.

In three cases involving elderly women with rheumatoid arthritis, doctors at Haywood Hospital in Stoke on Trent, England, administered 500 milligrams of vitamin C daily for an unspecified period. In all three cases, the bruising disappeared rapidly.

The researchers speculate that the vitamin C deficiencies in these three women were the result not only of poor nutrition but also of a peculiar combination of circumstances relating to the disease. The inflammation that characterizes rheumatoid arthritis tends to deplete the body's stores of vitamin C, and the drugs taken to combat inflammation — nonsteroidal anti-inflammatory preparations — interfere with vitamin C metabolism and excretion *(British Journal of Rheumatology).*

FISH OIL
MAY HELP DIABETICS

Omega-3 fatty acids—found in fish oil—are the latest darling of the nutrition community. And with good reason. Consumption of fish has been linked to good cardiovascular health, relief from migraine and prevention of breast cancer.

Now, Dutch researchers have found that by supplementing the diets of non-insulin-dependent diabetics with omega-3 fatty acids, they can actually improve the patients' sensitivity to their own insulin.

In the non-insulin-dependent diabetic, the pancreas produces insulin in amounts that vary from too little to too much to normal. But these patients, who frequently develop the disease because of obesity, tend to be insulin resistant, meaning their insulin is not as effective in regulating blood sugar.

The researchers concluded that supplementation with omega-3 fatty acids improved the effectiveness of insulin on the patients' blood sugar metabolism *(Netherlands Journal of Medicine)*.

GIVE YOUR GUMS ENOUGH "C"

There is new evidence that vitamin C may influence the early stages of gingivitis, a gum inflammation that frequently precedes full-blown gum disease, the major cause of tooth loss in adults.

Researchers at the School of Dentistry at the University of California's San Francisco campus found that gingivitis increased when volunteers were deprived of vitamin C for a time, then decreased significantly when their diets were supplemented with vitamin C.

The volunteers ate a diet that gave them all the nutrients they required except vitamin C. During the study's first two weeks, they received oral doses of 60 milligrams a day of vitamin C, the Recommended Dietary Allowance, to bring them all to the same baseline level. Then, in the following four weeks, they received a placebo (dummy pill) instead of the vitamin. For a three-week period after that, they received a 600-milligram dose followed by a four-week placebo period.

Though the volunteers showed no signs of serious gum disease during the period when they were vitamin C-deficient and, in fact, had no increase in the amount of the plaque that leads to gum disease, they did have far more inflammation and bleeding than in the periods when they were getting supplements. The bleeding and inflammation subsided significantly when they were taking vitamin C daily *(Journal of Periodontology)*.

FOLATE
FOR GINGIVITIS

Two studies have found that a topical treatment of folate, a B vitamin, may reduce the inflammation and soreness of gingivitis by increasing the resistance of gums to local irritants.

Researchers at the New Jersey Medical School and the School of Dentistry at the University of Otago in New Zealand both found that an oral rinse of folate was effective against this condition.

The New Jersey researchers thought of using folate against gingivitis because, in animal studies, folate deficiency was associated with generalized gum inflammation. Folate supplements given orally to humans, however, produced only minor improvements.

Since folate can be absorbed directly by the gums, the scientists administered a rinse to 15 subjects, who experienced a significant decrease in gum inflammation over 60 days.

The New Zealand researchers also found that the folate rinse was effective in treating gum inflammation, even that which occurs in pregnant women *(General Dentistry)*.

SMOKING, LUNG CANCER AND DIET

Not all smokers develop lung cancer. To find out if diet might offer some protection, researchers from Brigham and Women's Hospital and Harvard Medical School in Boston and Harvard School of Public Health, Cambridge, Massachusetts, reviewed studies comparing the intake of vitamin A, vitamin C and other nutrients in people who later developed cancer and those who remained healthy. These nutrients, because they are antioxidants, may halt damage to cells that can lead to cancer.

Answer: Those people whose intake of vitamin A from green and yellow vegetables was in the top 20 to 25 percent had about half the lung cancer risk of those in the lowest 20 to 25 percent. In one study, a strong protective effect was found in those who ate a green salad or fruit, including juice, five to seven times a week.

Few studies have been done in humans to explore a vitamin C and lung cancer link. Adding vitamin C has reversed malignant changes in hamster lung cells induced by tobacco smoke, but several other experiments have shown that even high levels of vitamin C supplementation have little effect on cancer.

Still the best advice: If you smoke, stop. "Cigarette smoking is the major known cause of lung cancer, and smoking cessation would be of more benefit than change in any other single behavior," conclude the researchers *(Archives of Internal Medicine)*.

VITAMIN B$_{12}$ AND THE ELDERLY

Old age is traditionally thought of as a time of decline, particularly when it comes to nutrition. Studies have shown that as a person ages, the levels of certain nutrients, notably vitamins C and B$_{12}$, tend to drop.

But a new study by a group of scientists at the University of Massachusetts Medical Center indicates that thought may be a little hasty. When they looked at the B$_{12}$ concentrations in a group of 179 volunteers between the ages of 20 and 93, they found no difference between the young and old.

Why such a dramatic departure from other reputable studies? The researchers theorize that in other studies, scientists relied on the most convenient populations—the institutionalized, who have a greater potential for vitamin deficiencies than normal, healthy, independent-living people. The Massachusetts study used the latter group, even winnowing out those people on medications, such as oral contraceptives, that have been associated with depressed blood B$_{12}$ levels.

They also suggest that the method of determining B$_{12}$ values in blood may be at fault. Some techniques have proved more reliable than others *(American Journal of Clinical Pathology)*.

EGGS NEEDN'T SCRAMBLE YOUR HEALTH

You *can* have your low blood cholesterol and eat your eggs, too, according to a recent study by British researchers. The trick is to stick to a diet fairly low in saturated fats but high in polyunsaturates and fiber.

In the study, participants ate either two or seven eggs a week for eight weeks. During that time, they were also on a low-fat, high-fiber diet.

The group eating seven eggs a week did see an initial early rise in blood cholesterol levels. But by the eighth week of the study, cholesterol levels in both groups had stabilized below prestudy levels. Researchers speculate that in the seven-egg group, body metabolism slowly adjusted to larger amounts of cholesterol.

The bottom line on eggs? Researchers at a recent conference sponsored by the Egg Nutrition Center say it's this: A heart-healthy diet can include a few eggs a week. Just make sure they're not coddled in butter.

BONES ARE STRONGER WITH VITAMIN C

Aging bones can become almost as weak and crumbly—and as unreliable a support—as a termite-infested rafter. But now a group of British researchers think vitamin C may help stop this process.

In a recent study, they found very low blood levels of vitamin C in patients with hip fractures compared to people without fractures—even when hipbone calcium content was the same.

It's known that, within the bone, vitamin C is needed by an enzyme (prolylhydroxylase) to create a spiderweb of connective tissue. It's on this framework of tissue that bone-hardening calcium is laid. So without adequate vitamin C, bones can't use calcium.

Severe vitamin C deficiencies are rare, but they're more likely to be found in older people living alone, says Beverly Peterkofsky, Ph.D., a National Institutes of Health biochemist. "Healthy bones are just one more reason older people should make sure they're eating plenty of vitamin C-rich fresh fruits and vegetables."

HEAVY DRINKING
HOISTS STROKE RISK

"Heavy alcohol consumption is an important and underrecognized independent risk factor for stroke in men," concluded a team of British researchers. They examined the drinking habits of 230 people admitted to a Birmingham hospital for stroke as compared with those of 230 patients admitted to the same hospital for other reasons (but who were of the same age, sex and race as the stroke victims).

Their conclusion: "Among men, the relative risk of stroke . . . was lower in light drinkers (those consuming 10 to 90 grams of alcohol weekly) than in nondrinkers . . . but was four times higher in heavy drinkers (more than 300 grams weekly) than in nondrinkers."

Since ten grams is roughly equivalent to a single drink, putting away more than four drinks a day would put you in this high-risk group. Light alcohol consumption actually seemed to *reduce* the men's stroke risk slightly. Interestingly enough, this is the same "J-shaped curve" of relative risk that's been noted in high blood pressure. Teetotalers are actually at slightly higher risk of having high blood pressure than moderate drinkers, but heavy drinkers are at the highest risk of all *(New England Journal of Medicine)*.

GOOD NEWS
FOR SHELLFISH LOVERS

Due to their reputed high cholesterol content, shellfish have long been taboo for people on low-cholesterol diets. Now researchers have found that the cholesterol content of mollusks — like clams, oysters and scallops — is considerably lower than was once believed.

William Conner, M.D., of the Oregon Health Sciences University in Portland, found that feeding healthy men approximately one pound of shellfish (a combo of either clams, oysters and scallops or crab, shrimp and lobster) didn't significantly raise their blood cholesterol levels.

Crab, lobster and shrimp are higher in cholesterol content than mollusks, yet eating even a pound of these foods raised cholesterol levels only slightly in healthy men, the Oregon researchers found.

Another bonus: Shellfish are low in fat and contain omega-3 fatty acids, which are thought to combat heart disease. The (new) bottom line: "It would appear that shrimp [as well as other shellfish] can be included in the diets of patients [with high cholesterol levels] on an occasional basis" *(Journal of the American Medical Association).*

The Healing Power of Nutrition

Regenerate Your Health with Better Nutrition

By Robert Rodale, Editor, *Prevention*® magazine

Food is fuel for the body, nothing more. That's how most people think of nutrition.

But consider this radical idea: What you eat is more than merely sustaining—it can be regenerating. And I mean regenerating in ways that most people haven't even considered, ways that scientists are just now beginning to understand.

Nutrients—vitamins, minerals, protein, carbohydrates and the like—nourish flesh, blood and bone. But in the right amounts, in the proper combinations, they also have the power to renew the body, repair physical damage, prevent the onset of disease and maybe even reverse some of the signs of aging.

When you realize this—that supplying yourself with the proper nutrients can foster growth and renewal—you're thinking "regenerative nutrition." And just *thinking* in these terms can give you a big push down the road to well-being.

To me, regeneration (which can apply to economics, agriculture and other fields, as well as nutrition) means changing or reforming for the better by using your own resources. So in regenerative agriculture, for example, farmers thrive by planting legumes that pull nitrogen from the air and into the soil, instead of buying expensive synthetic nitrogen fertilizers. In regenerative economics, communities produce locally most of the consumer products they need rather than paying higher

19

prices for goods produced elsewhere. And in regenerative nutrition, you enhance, even renew, your health by taking charge of it, by manipulating your nutrient intake, a potent personal resource.

The body responds to regenerative nutrition because it's already preoccupied with regeneration. It's a pulsing, humming mass of regenerative processes—cells replace cells, tissues heal, muscles expand, nerves and organs change to meet new biological demands. So regenerative nutrition (like exercise, weight control, preventive dentistry and other regenerating strategies) is a way of turning up the body's existing regenerative power.

Scientists dream of regenerating human organs. With a disdainful look toward immortality schemes and myths of eternal youth, I dream of finding ways to regenerate the whole person, body and soul, starting with techniques for helping the body do what it does best. Just sharing such a dream can be renewing in itself, an inspirational nudge toward better health.

Regenerating Bodies

Inch by inch, scientists are documenting the nutritional road to regeneration. So far, they've found at least three ways that nutrition can regenerate you.

Reversing Deficiencies ● When you don't get enough vitamins and minerals over a long period of time, your body literally degenerates. Without enough vitamin A, you get skin problems, greater susceptibility to infection, eye trouble, even blindness. Without enough B vitamins, you're open to fatigue, nerve damage, poor memory, sleep problems, anorexia, anemia.

The catalog of physical degeneration caused by lack of nutrients is long and familiar. What isn't so well appreciated is that getting enough of the right nutrients can halt the decay and often put it in reverse. The body proves for itself that the opposite of degeneration is regeneration.

Reversing Excesses ● Have you ever talked to someone who survived a heart attack, then changed the way he ate to forestall a second coronary? Some of these survivors may tell you how great they feel since they started cutting down on fat, alcohol, sugar, salt and cholesterol. They may say things like, "I feel like a brand-new person," or "I never felt better in my life."

Such dramatic testimonies are affidavits of nutritional regeneration. You hear them from people battling weight problems, diabetes, allergies, fatigue and other maladies. You even hear them from people who have no known ailments at all. The words of renewal echo what scientists have already verified in test tube and clinic: Eliminating dietary excesses can give your body a chance to heal, even feel young again.

Slowing the Clock ● Scientists have been presenting evidence suggesting that it may be possible to use certain nutrients to affect aspects of the aging process. There are intriguing but unconfirmed studies showing that people who had higher intakes of certain vitamins outlived people who had lower intakes. And there's also very preliminary evidence that antioxidants like vitamin E may be able to prevent the aging of certain cells. (Whether vitamin E can actually increase the life span of humans has yet to be determined scientifically.)

The most impressive research yet shows that nutrients may be able to prevent or reverse some disorders associated with getting old. Vitamin D and calcium may slow down the bone-degenerating disease known as osteoporosis. Vitamin E may relieve the circulation problem called intermittent claudication. Vitamins C and A may boost immunity. These and other healing possibilities are the first sketchy signs that nutrition may be able to de-age the aging body.

Internal and External

By far the greatest advantage of nutritional regeneration is that it can provide what I call "low-input solutions" to health problems.

By "low-input" I mean low-cost—inexpensive in money, energy or time. If a treatment or preventive is low input, it must be regenerative. For, by definition, regenerative health solutions are inexpensive, readily available and abundant. They have to be: They come mostly from internal resources we already own, resources that generally grow as we grow.

High-input answers to health troubles, on the other hand,

have external sources and are therefore costly and often scarce. They're usually medical—which means professionally administered (often with high-tech hardware) and sometimes hard on the body (as surgery or drugs with severe side effects are).

Let's say you have the painful wrist and hand disorder called carpal tunnel syndrome. One high-input external solution to the problem (if anti-inflammatory medications or cortisone injections fail) is surgery—which may cost hundreds of dollars, may require a lot of time in convalescence and still may not correct the problem. A reported low-input solution for some people is vitamin B_6. Preliminary research shows that some victims of carpal tunnel syndrome have found relief from symptoms after taking daily doses of B_6 for several months.

Here's an even more dramatic example: cancer. The high-input answer to this scourge is chemotherapy, radiation treatments, surgery, drugs. Only victims of cancer know—in many painful ways—how truly costly these therapies can be. Scientists, though, are working on proving the power of a low-input nutritional solution: prevention of cancer with green and yellow vegetables and fruit.

Studies from all over the world suggest that there's something in these edibles (possibly beta-carotene) that reduces your risk of several types of cancer. A Harvard University study, for example, found that people who reported the highest consumption of carrots, squash, tomatoes, salads or leafy greens, dried fruits, fresh strawberries or melon, broccoli or brussels sprouts had a decreased risk of cancer. This and other evidence prompted the National Academy of Sciences to ask Americans to start eating more vegetables.

Everyone has heard about the high-tech approaches to heart disease—bypass surgery, heart transplants, artificial hearts. As necessary as these may be in certain cases, their cost in dollars, risk and pain is enormous.

According to a growing body of evidence, a low-input nutritional alternative to such last-ditch measures might be fish and fish oil. They contain unsaturated fats that apparently can lower cholesterol, reduce triglycerides (another blood fat) and help reduce the chances of blood clots that can cause strokes and heart attacks. In other words, the simple act of adding more fish or fish oil to your diet may reduce your risk of getting heart disease in the first place.

Does all this mean that high-input external sources are never appropriate? That low-input regenerative solutions should always be preferred when there's a choice? Of course not. Well-being is always a matter of balancing the regenerative internal strategies with the external.

The point is not to waste our own regenerative power but to use it to best advantage. My guess is that if we start thinking regenerative nutrition, we'll start doing regenerative nutrition. And that just might set the scales in better balance, a notch or two closer to regenerative living.

Your Lunch Can Crunch Disease

What manic mind could have guessed that one of the great instruments against 20th-century disease would turn out to be something as simple as, well, your lunch?

It's true. Science is discovering that food is not just fodder, but a force—a force for promoting or preventing illness. Some researchers, for example, estimate that poor dietary habits are responsible for 30 to 40 percent of cancers in men and 60 percent of cancers in women. And others say that simply changing the way we eat could avert many cancer deaths. Diet has also been recruited in the war against heart disease, osteoporosis (the bone-thinning malady), high blood pressure and other disorders. And some researchers are predicting that certain elements in food may become more potent disease fighters than either scalpels or pills.

Here's the latest news from the new science of protective nutrition.

Olive Oil against Cholesterol

THE PROBLEM: With the certitude that comes from solid research, scientists have accused cholesterol of causing heart disease. They now know that too much cholesterol and saturated fat in the diet dumps too much cholesterol in the blood—a biochemical overload that can slowly choke off arteries, as lime clogs plumbing.

THE NEW RESEARCH: In the dietary war on cholesterol, there's been the good (polyunsaturated oils), the bad (saturated fats) and the neutral (monounsaturated oils). The polyunsaturates (predominant in safflower, corn and other vegetable oils) lower cholesterol levels. Saturated fats (found in meats, butter and egg yolks) raise them. And monounsaturates (predominant in olive oil and nuts) are supposed to stay out of the fray.

But now there's evidence that the monounsaturates may not be bystanders at all, but tough troops against cholesterol—maybe even tougher than the polyunsaturates.

This news comes from researcher Scott M. Grundy, M.D., Ph.D., director of the Center for Human Nutrition of the University of Texas Health Science Center in Dallas, and a colleague. They devised three different liquid diets, each containing either saturated, polyunsaturated or monounsaturated oils but all providing 40 percent of the calories as fat. They gave the diets to 20 patients, letting them stay on each diet for four weeks, and monitored their cholesterol levels.

The results: The monounsaturated diet was just as effective as the polyunsaturated diet in lowering both total cholesterol and LDL (low-density lipoprotein) cholesterol (the most harmful type). And there was promising (but not conclusive) evidence that the monounsaturated diet reduced HDL (high-density lipoprotein) cholesterol (the protective type) less.

"We knew that the rate of cardiovascular disease was very low in the Mediterranean region, where people cook primarily with olive oil," says Dr. Grundy. "Unfortunately, a thorough clinical comparison of monounsaturates and polyunsaturates had not been made, so no one knew whether monounsaturates lowered cholesterol levels as effectively. We now know they do."

THE IMPLICATIONS: Olive oil and peanut oil (prime sources of monounsaturates) may deserve a lot more space in most diets.

Dr. Grundy recommends a low-fat diet with less than 10 percent of calories in saturated fat, 5 to 10 percent in polyunsaturates and 10 to 15 percent in monounsaturates.

Calcium against Colon Cancer

THE PROBLEM: Colorectal cancer is the second deadliest cancer in the nation, killing about 60,000 people a year. (Lung cancer is number one, felling about 126,000 a year.)

THE NEW RESEARCH: Among scientists, there's a growing suspicion that manipulating certain factors in the diet may help prevent colorectal cancer. Two such promising factors tested by medical detectives are lowered dietary fat and increased fiber, and now researchers are looking at a new preventive possibility: calcium.

The idea that calcium might help deter colon cancer got a boost when researchers noticed that the disease seemed to strike more frequently in latitudes far from the equator—places with less sunshine. The hypothesis was that since sunlight helps the body make vitamin D, and vitamin D enables the body to absorb calcium, it was this nutritional pair that reduced colon cancer.

On top of this, scientists reported that in Scandinavia, colon cancer occurs least where consumption of milk is greatest. And a 19-year study in Chicago revealed that men with the lowest intake of vitamin D and calcium had about three times the risk of colorectal cancer as those who had the highest intake.

The latest word comes from researchers at Memorial Sloan-Kettering Cancer Center and Cornell University Medical College in New York City. They gave daily doses of 1,250 milligrams of calcium to people with family histories of colon cancer. The idea was to discover what effect the calcium might have on excessive proliferation (duplication) of cells in the lining of the colon. Excessive proliferation is often found in people prone to developing colon cancer. The researchers reported that before the calcium supplements were taken, cell proliferation was just what you'd expect in people susceptible to colon cancer, but that after two to three months of taking

calcium, proliferation was lower—comparable to that of people with a lower risk of colon cancer. "Calcium modifies the
environment in the colon," says chief researcher Martin Lipkin,
M.D. "We think that calcium binds [captures] bile and fatty
acids, reducing their irritation to the colon lining and thus
decreasing the proliferation of cells. The result is a lower risk
of colon cancer."

THE IMPLICATIONS: "We intend to conduct more research
on calcium and colon cancer," says Dr. Lipkin. "We want to
see what effect calcium might have on ulcerative colitis, familial polyposis and other conditions that may lead to cancer of
the colon."

Low-Fat Diets and High Blood Pressure

THE PROBLEM: High blood pressure is a major risk factor
for stroke, coronary heart disease, kidney failure and other
woes. Over 57 million Americans have it, and almost half of
them don't even know it.

THE NEW RESEARCH: Thanks to years of scientific
spadework, we know that in some people too much salt (or
rather the sodium in it) instigates high blood pressure.

But now comes news that salt may not be the only dietary
wild card in hypertension. There's mounting evidence that
dietary fat can have an effect on blood pressure, too.

A recent study—the latest in a long line of similar
investigations—suggests that it may actually be possible for
people to lower their blood pressure by cutting back on (or
changing the type of) fat in their diet. In the three-month trial,
middle-aged men with normal blood pressure followed either
a low-fat diet (25 percent of calories from fat; equal amounts
of polyunsaturated and saturated fats) or a more typically
American diet (about 40 percent of calories from fat, mostly
saturated). They all consumed the same kinds of foods, but
the low-fat group ate leaner fare—like meat trimmed of fat,
low-fat milk and margarine. And in line with the results of
other studies, there was a 9 percent drop in blood pressure in
the group that was on the low-fat diet.

Researcher James M. Iacono, Ph.D., director of the U.S.
Department of Agriculture's Western Human Nutrition Research

50 SUPER FOODS

that can help lower your risk of . . .

Cardio-vascular problems	Cancer	Osteo-porosis	Hyper-tension
Almonds	Apples	Broccoli	Apples
Avocados	Apricots	Buttermilk	Asparagus
Cashews	Bananas	Dandelion	Bananas
Hazel nuts	Beans, baked	greens	Beans, kidney
Herring,	Beans, kidney	Milk, skim	Broccoli
Atlantic	Blackberries	Molasses,	Cabbage
Mackerel,	Broccoli	blackstrap	Cantaloupe
Atlantic	Buttermilk	Salmon, pink	Cauliflower
Olive oil	Cabbage	(with	Eggplant
Pecans	Cantaloupe	bones)	Grapefruit
Pistachios	Carrots	Sardines	Honeydew
Salmon, pink	Cereals,	Yogurt,	melon
Trout,	high-fiber	low-fat	Nectarines
rainbow	Collards		Orange juice
Tuna	Dandelion		Peas, green
	greens		Potatoes
	Endive, raw		Prunes
	Kale		Raisins
	Milk, skim		Squash
	Molasses,		Sweet
	blackstrap		potatoes
	Mustard		Watermelon
	greens		
	Salmon, pink		
	Sardines		
	Spinach		
	Squash		
	Sweet		
	potatoes		
	Watermelon		
	Yogurt,		
	low-fat		

Center in San Francisco, says that the data he gathered suggest a cause for the decrease in blood pressure. "The bodies of the men in the low-fat group excreted [got rid of] 4 percent more sodium and 11 percent more potassium that those in the normal-fat group," he says. "The excretion of these two minerals, one of which is known to sometimes raise blood pressure with higher daily intake, may be what triggers the reductions in blood pressure."

THE IMPLICATIONS: If such low-fat diets can pull down blood pressure as well as research suggests, they may soon become as crucial as low-salt eating in the nondrug treatment of hypertension. "Until scientists can define the most effective low-fat diet for reducing blood pressure," says Dr. Iacono, "the wisest approach is to follow the current recommendations: Reduce overall fat to about 30 percent of total calories and maintain equal amounts of polyunsaturated and saturated fats."

Fish and Fish Oil for Heart Disease

THE PROBLEM: Heart disease, in all its dire variations, is the nations's most efficient executioner, killing more people than accidents, cancer, suicide or even murder.

THE NEW RESEARCH: Headlines have been announcing what study after study has been showing. Fish and fish oil are true friends of the heart.

It's now established that the oil in many fish contains large amounts of unsaturated fats called omega-3 fatty acids and that these "good fats" are experts at helping to protect your heart and blood vessels. There's evidence that omega-3's can lower cholesterol, reduce triglycerides (another blood fat considered a risk factor for heart disease) and help cut the likelihood of blood clots that can cause strokes and heart attacks.

The evidence for the positive power of omega-3 is so impressive that scientists from around the world suggested at a recent conference that people could reduce their risk of chronic illnesses (including heart disease, arthritis, cancer and others) if they included more fish or fish oil in their diets. And the National Institutes of Health (NIH) are launching major research into the effect of fish and fish oils on health and disease (including heart disorders).

The latest studies corroborate omega-3's good reputation. One of them was conducted by Sanford E. Warren, M.D., of Beth Israel Hospital in Boston, and his colleagues. They report that after they gave daily doses of cod-liver oil (which contains omega-3 fatty acids) to seven heart patients, the patients experienced improvements in blood lipid chemistries. (Because cod-liver oil contains large amounts of vitamins A and D, which can be toxic in high doses, you shouldn't take more than one tablespoon a day without consulting your doctor.) The four men and three women had increases in beneficial HDL cholesterol, favorable shifts in the ratio of total cholesterol to HDL (a predictor of heart disease) and indications that their arteries may be less likely to clog or develop blood clots.

THE IMPLICATIONS: Prodded by the omega-3 research, some medical authorities have issued timely advice: Eat more fish! Most investigators think that as few as two to four fish meals a week might be sufficient to exert a positive effect. "Americans eat an average of one fish meal per week," says Artemis Simopoulos, M.D., former chairperson of the NIH Nutrition Coordinating Commitee. "The idea is to raise this to at least two fish meals a week."

Fat and Breast Cancer

THE PROBLEM: Breast cancer is a major cancer killer of American women, and among those aged 40 to 44 it causes more deaths than anything else.

THE NEW RESEARCH: In 1942 a scientist demonstrated that there's a probable link between breast cancer and fat in the diet. And the evidence for that link has been getting stronger—and more complex—ever since. Now it seems clear that the more fat you have in your diet, the more likely you are to get breast cancer.

But there are some new wrinkles in the data.

There's accumulating evidence that a low-fat diet may actually prolong the lives of women who already have breast cancer. In a recent study of 953 women with breast cancer, researchers discovered that the women's risk of death increased 1.4 times for every 1,000 grams of fat eaten per month (equivalent to one extra pat of butter or margarine per day). This connection between life expectancy and fat intake was especially strong for women with cancers that were spreading.

Echoing the reports of other scientists, researcher Rashida Karmali, Ph.D., of Rutgers University, New Brunswick, New

Jersey, and her colleagues say that they were able to protect laboratory rats against breast cancer by feeding them fish oil. "Fish oil," says Dr. Karmali, "inhibited the growth of transplanted tumors, helped block development of chemically induced tumors and lowered levels of a biochemical indicator of cancer activity." Preventing cancer in rats is a long way from preventing it in people, she says. But these preliminary findings hint at promising possibilities.

THE IMPLICATIONS: Do scientists now have enough information to devise a diet that prevents breast cancer, a diet including the right dietary fats in specific amounts?

Not yet. So far all they know is that cutting overall fat intake is likely to reduce the risk of breast cancer. Says the National Research Council: To lower the risk of this disease and colon cancer, pare down dietary fat to 30 percent of total calories. "Indeed," the council admits, "the data could be used to justify an even greater reduction."

Calcium versus Osteoporosis

THE PROBLEM: Osteoporosis thins bone throughout the body—slowly, silently draining the skeleton of strength until it cracks. The disease is epidemic in America, especially among older women, leading to 210,000 hip fractures a year and 30,000 deaths.

THE NEW RESEARCH: Scientists have reported that calcium supplements are likely to help slow down bone loss and thus put the brakes on osteoporosis. That's why so may doctors prescribe calcium (up to 1,000 milligrams) to patients with the disease, along with vitamin D (400 international units), estrogen, exercise and fluoride.

But there's been precious little evidence that calcium supplements could actually help reverse bone loss—until now.

In a study conducted by Paul D. Miller, M.D., of the University of Colorado School of Medicine in Denver, 21 patients with osteoporosis actually gained bone mass after a year of taking daily doses of 1,500 to 2,000 milligrams of calcium plus vitamin D.

In fact, by the end of the year, their bones had returned to normal mass. And instead of showing a continuing decline in mass, the bones of another 29 patients showed no change.

Dr. Miller reports that the calcium and vitamin D therapy seemed to work for some women regardless of whether they took estrogen. And taking fluoride along with the nutrients didn't seem to have any effect on bone loss at all.

"The increase in bone mass was very unusual," says Dr. Miller. "We are quite excited about the apparent reversibility of osteoporosis."

THE IMPLICATIONS: Up to now, osteoporosis has been regarded as merely treatable, not curable. But if Dr. Miller's findings are corroborated by other research, calcium (with vitamin D) may emerge as the core ingredient in a long-awaited cure.

Until then, we can heed current advice from a growing medical consensus: Make sure you're getting enough calcium.

A committee of scientists from the National Institutes of Health says that after menopause, women should get 1,500 milligrams of calcium per day; before menopause, they should get 1,000 to 1,500 milligrams per day.

In addition to taking calcium and vitamin D, experts say, women who want to avert osteoporosis should avoid smoking and excessive alcohol, eat a balanced diet, get regular exercise like walking and shun heavy intake of caffeine.

HEALTHY MENU MAKEOVERS

Thanks to the new science of protective nutrition, we now know that some foods are more likely to keep you healthy than others, that some meals are good disease preventives and others are bad medicine. The menus on the following pages can help you tell which is which and show you how to exchange one for the other.

Menu one is a nutritional hazard—too many risks (fat, sodium and cholesterol) and not enough safety features (calcium, fiber, monounsaturated fats, omega-3 fatty acids, vitamin A). Menu two is a slight improvement. Menu three is even better. And menu four is nearly ideal—very low in the risky ingredients and very high in the protective ones.

DISASTER

Breakfast
2 fried eggs
3 strips bacon
2 slices toasted white bread
1 pat butter
1 cup coffee
1 tbsp. nondairy creamer
4 oz. apple juice

Lunch
2 pieces fried chicken
 (drumstick and thigh)
3½ oz. french fries
½ cup coleslaw
12 oz. cola

Dinner
Lettuce wedge (¼ head)
1 tablespoon Russian
 dressing
6¼ oz. spareribs, braised
 with BBQ sauce
½ cup Spanish rice
½ cup boiled green beans
1 slice cheesecake with
 cherry sauce
1 cup coffee
1 tbsp. nondairy creamer

Percentage of total calories in fat: 51%
Percentage of total calories in monounsaturated fat: 0.5%
Cholesterol: 912 mg.
Sodium: 3,771 mg.
Calcium: 476 mg.
Omega-3 fatty acids: 0 g.
Vitamin A: 3,913 I.U.

BORDERLINE

Breakfast

1 poached egg
2 slices toasted rye bread
1 pat margarine
1 cup coffee
1 tbsp. whole milk
4 oz. grape juice

Lunch

4 oz. chicken salad on
  croissant
1 cup marinated vegetables
12 oz. lemonade

Dinner

Tossed salad (1 cup lettuce,
  3 tomato wedges, 3
  cucumber slices)
1 tbsp. buttermilk dressing
4 oz. breaded, fried
  haddock
½ cup buttered carrots
½ cup mashed potatoes
1 pat margarine
1 slice angel food cake
1 cup coffee
1 tbsp. whole milk

Percentage of total calories in fat: 43%
Percentage of total calories in monounsaturated fat: 13%
Cholesterol: 350 mg.
Sodium: 2,663 mg.
Calcium: 424 mg.
Omega-3 fatty acids: 0.2 g.
Vitamin A: 25,244 I.U.

ABOVE AVERAGE

Breakfast

3 whole wheat buttermilk
  pancakes

1 tbsp. maple syrup

1 pat margarine

1 poached pear

1 cup coffee

1 tbsp. 2% milk

4 oz. apricot nectar

Lunch

1 cup homemade vegetable
  soup

4 oz. tuna salad on whole
  wheat roll

6 oz. baked steak fries

1 cup apple juice

Dinner

1 cup spinach salad with
  mushrooms

1 tbsp. olive oil and
  vinegar dressing

1 serving vegetarian
  lasagna

1 serving brussels sprouts
  in mustard sauce

1 slice whole wheat Italian
  bread

1 tsp. garlic spread

1 baked apple

1 cup coffee

1 tbsp. 2% milk

Percentage of total calories in fat: 28%
Percentage of total calories in monounsaturated fat: 10%
Cholesterol: 224 mg.
Sodium: 3,339 mg.
Calcium: 1,360 mg.
Omega-3 fatty acids: 0.45 g.
Vitamin A: 11,329 I.U.

MAXIMUM PROTECTION

Breakfast

2 oat bran muffins

1 tbsp. fruit butter

1 cup plain low-fat yogurt
with ½ cup fresh
strawberries

1 cup decaf coffee

1 tbsp. skim milk

4 oz. orange juice

Lunch

1 serving vegetarian chili

1 piece cornbread

1 tsp. soft margarine

1 cup tossed salad (loose-
leaf lettuce, beet greens,
grated carrot, red
cabbage, parsley)

1 tbsp. Italian dressing,
made with olive oil and
fresh herbs

1 cup skim milk

Dinner

1 cup watercress and
romaine lettuce

1 tbsp. tomato vinaigrette
dressing

4 oz. broiled salmon steak

½ cup steamed broccoli
with toasted almonds

1 serving brown rice pilaf

1 cup melon-ball fruit salad

1 cup decaf coffee

1 tbsp. skim milk

Percentage of total calories in fat: 29%
Percentage of total calories in monounsaturated fat: 9%
Cholesterol: 112 mg.
Sodium: 1,028 mg.
Calcium: 1,331 mg.
Omega-3 fatty acids: 1.6 g.
Vitamin A: 16,780 I.U.

YOUR LIBRARY
OF PROTECTIVE NUTRITION

The following books are recommended reading for anyone who wants to know more about deterring disease through healthy eating and cooking.

• *The Lifelong Nutrition Guide,* by Brian L. G. Morgan, Ph.D. (New York: Prentice-Hall, 1983. 207 pages). A comprehensive handbook on eating for health at each stage of your life. It shows you how to customize a risk-reducing diet for your personal needs. Includes chapters on vitamins, minerals, exercise, heart disease, cancer, obesity, child nutrition and aging.

• *The Rutgers Guide to Lowering Your Cholesterol,* by Hans Fisher, Ph.D., and Eugene Boe (New Brunswick, N.J.: Rutgers University Press, 1985. 218 pages). A clear-headed analysis of how cholesterol instigates heart disease and how to stop it through smart nutrition, exercise and other strategies. Includes an anticholesterol meal plan, low-cholesterol recipes and tips on how to distinguish the foods that fight and invite high blood levels of cholesterol.

• *Food and Nutrition,* by Nancy Nugent and the editors of *Prevention* magazine (Emmaus, Pa.: Rodale Press, 1983. 168 pages). An easy-to-use guide to putting the facts of preventive nutrition to work in everyday life. Shows you how to select, buy, preserve and enjoy the freshest and most nutritious foods—without wasting time or money. Includes information on kitchen tools and techniques, healthful dining out and snacking and nutrition-wise gardening. Part of the 14-book series, The Prevention Total Health System®.

• *The Living Heart Diet,* by Michael E. Debakey, M.D., et al. (New York: Raven Press, 1984. 397 pages). A thorough review of current knowledge about heart disease (what it is, what causes it) and how to prevent or treat it through nutrition. Presents a medically tested healthy-heart diet and variations of it for specific needs (low calorie, low sodium, diabetic and others). Includes menus, over 500 recipes, questionnaires that reveal your attitudes toward eating, tips on healthy dining away from home and an 11-step plan for safely losing weight.

YOUR LIBRARY
OF PROTECTIVE NUTRITION
— *Continued*

• *Planning Meals That Lower Cancer Risk: A Reference Guide,* from the American Institute for Cancer Research (Washington, D.C.: American Institute for Cancer Research, 1984. 88 pages). An authoritative handbook on how to create meals that follow the anticancer guidelines from the National Academy of Sciences. Includes information on how to reconcile your dietary needs and personal food preferences with the guidelines, practical tips on getting more fiber and less fat in your diet, menus and recipes.

• *The Calcium Bible: How to Have Better Bones All Your Life,* by Patricia Hausman (New York: Rawson Associates, 1985. 205 pages). A reliable review of the latest calcium research and what it means to your health. Includes a quiz that reveals how much calcium your diet contains, recommendations on how much of the bone-building nutrients you need during each stage of your life, guidelines for selecting calcium supplements, a list of 300 calcium-rich foods and tips on getting calcium into special diets.

• *Healthy Cooking,* by Sharon Claessens (Emmaus, Pa.: Rodale Press, 1984. 168 pages). A practical guide to the art of preparing food that's kind to body, soul and palate—high in taste, nutrients and fiber and low in salt, fat, cholesterol and sugar. Features expert instruction and scores of recipes for creating soups and stews, breads and rolls, seafood dishes, hors d'oeuvres, vegetarian feasts, side dishes, desserts, beverages, meat and poultry dishes and salads. Part of The Prevention Total Health System®.

• *The New American Diet,* by Sonja L. Connor, R.D., and William E. Connor, M.D. (New York: Simon & Schuster, 1986. 410 pages). This is the handbook of a scientifically designed and "people-tested" diet to help prevent heart disease, stroke, hypertension, obesity, several kinds of cancer and other disorders. It shows you how to slowly phase in the diet over several years without sacrificing taste or restricting calories. Includes nearly 350 recipes drawn from all over the world.

More Fish,
Less Arthritis Pain

The advice to "take your medicine with your meal" might someday change to "your medicine *is* your meal"—if the meal is fish and you have arthritis.

Daily doses of fish oil, which contains omega-3 fatty acids, led to modest but significant improvement in the symptoms of rheumatoid arthritis patients studied recently at Harvard Medical School and Albany (New York) Medical College.

These efforts are the first to show definite clinical effects of fish oil on an inflammatory disease. Previous work showing favorable results had been done on mice. These latest findings have prompted the National Institutes of Health to get additional clinical studies under way.

"Our trial, although it was relatively small, shows evidence that fish oil does have promise for inflammatory disease," says Richard I. Sperling, M.D., a Harvard University instructor of medicine.

Dr. Sperling's study targeted the biochemical aspect of fish oil in the body. Earlier, he and his colleagues looked at the cells of people who did not have inflammatory disease. Fish oil was added to their diets, and their cells were later examined to see if the fish oil could inhibit the ability of these cells to generate what researchers call "inflammatory products."

One such product thought to cause or contribute to the painful swelling of arthritis is leukotriene B4. At the end of Dr. Sperling's initial study, the added fish oil in the patients' diets seemed to result in significantly less leukotriene B4 production, and a small increase in the generation of a less inflammatory substance, leukotriene B5.

Fewer Tender Joints

The second step for the Harvard team was to repeat the trial with cells from 12 patients with active arthritis. "We saw the same thing in the diseased state—a suppression of inflammatory products," Dr. Sperling explains. "And the patients definitely felt better. They had fewer tender joints and reported less pain.

"Granted, we didn't have the placebo and double-blind study [where neither patients nor researchers know who's taking the active substance or a harmless, blank pill until the trial's end], so we can't say, 'Without a doubt, fish oil works, we proved it,'" he notes. "But other studies are going to follow this up, and right now we know we can at least biochemically alter the generation of inflammatory products in cells."

The other recent study was also encouraging. Thirty-three rheumatoid arthritis patients in an Albany Medical College trial took either 15 fish-oil capsules daily or a placebo, both in addition to their usual diet. They did this for 14 weeks, then all went through a four-week washout period (the fish oil or placebo was eliminated). At the end of the washout, patients received the opposite treatment for another 14 weeks and finished with a second washout.

The good news: an improved condition for patients while they were getting the fish oil. "They weren't in as much pain, their joints were less tender and they made it through the day longer before fatigue set in," says the study's leader, Joel M. Kremer, M.D., associate professor of medicine. "We also found benefits four weeks after the fish oil was discontinued," he adds.

Fishing for More Answers

Both Dr. Sperling and Dr. Kremer note that more research must back their early findings before any new recommendations on adding fish or fish-oil supplements to the diet are made with a higher degree of confidence.

In the meantime, "It's irrefutable that eating more fish is a healthy step for any person, arthritis or not," says Dr. Kremer. "Researchers do have more well-developed evidence that fish oil can be a key step in lowering cholesterol and fighting cardiovascular trouble such as atherosclerosis and heart attacks.

"In our studies, the doses of fish oil given were roughly equal to a salmon dinner or a can of sardines," Dr. Kremer explains.

"If you've got arthritis now," says Dr. Sperling, "you can use traditional therapies for relief and also continue to eat more fish. It certainly won't hurt, and it may help your inflammation."

Look for results of the National Institutes of Health studies sometime in the future. "Then," Dr. Sperling says, "look to the next few years for a possible new inflammatory disease treatment—fish oil."

How to Get Calcium into *Your* Bones

Unless you've been doing time in a Tibetan monastery, you've probably heard reports of how important calcium is for healthy bones. It's the element that keeps us standing tall, even as we age.

You may know calcium's benefits, but do you know how much calcium you're actually getting? And how to get as much as you need? Dietitians say most people have little idea how much calcium is in the foods they eat. And that they're unlikely to know that the Recommended Dietary Allowance (RDA) is

---

QUICK CALCIUM CALCULATIONS

Here's a simple way to determine how much calcium you're getting from food.

Any one of the following will give you about 300 milligrams of calcium: 8 ounces of skim, low-fat or whole milk or buttermilk; 1½ ounces of hard cheese; 1 cup of yogurt; 1½ slices of processed cheese; 2 cups of cottage cheese; 2 cups of ice milk or ice cream; 4 to 5 ounces of salmon (with bones); 3 ounces of sardines (with bones); 8 ounces of tofu (made with a calcium coagulant).

For a rough estimate of your daily intake, figure that three to four servings a day of any of these foods will put you into the 900- to 1,200-milligram range. The Recommended Dietary Allowance for calcium is 800 milligrams, although it's suggested that women get 1,000 to 1,500 milligrams a day to ward off osteoporosis.

---

800 milligrams for adults or that the National Institutes of Health recommend 1,000 milligrams daily for premenopausal women and 1,500 milligrams daily for postmenopausal women. Most people simply have no way of telling if their daily intake is adequate.

The following examples should help you to evaluate and, if necessary, correct your own diet. In many cases, simple changes in food choices are all that's needed. Where that's not possible, it's important to know how much additional calcium you may need as a supplement.

Perpetual Dieters

If you're trying to lose weight to improve your health, the last thing you want to do is cause a new health problem in the process.

"My experience is that people who are dieting are so wrapped up in losing weight that they don't pay attention to nutrient needs," says Patricia Hausman, nutritionist and author of *The Calcium Bible.* "They have to make a conscious effort if they are to get the calcium they need."

There are plenty of low-fat, low-calorie, calcium-rich foods. "If they have at least three glasses of skim milk a day, they're doing reasonably well," Hausman says. Each cup has about 300 milligrams of calcium. Or dieters can dig into bok choy, broccoli or kale, or collard, mustard or turnip greens. One cup of any of these vegetables (cooked) provides at least 100 milligrams of calcium and less than 50 calories.

Some cheeses are fairly low in calories. One ounce of mozzarella or provolone has more than 100 milligrams of calcium and about 100 calories. A half cup of 1 percent fat cottage cheese has 70 milligrams of calcium and 82 calories. The same amount of part-skim ricotta has 340 milligrams of calcium. Unfortunately, it also has 171 calories. A cup of nonfat yogurt has 450 milligrams of calcium and 125 calories. Canned salmon (be sure to eat those soft little bones!), shrimp and oysters are also delicious, low-calorie sources of calcium.

If you find that your diet simply isn't adding up, and you're not willing to make the dietary changes that boost calcium, consider adding supplements. The most common forms are calcium carbonate, calcium lactate, calcium gluconate, dicalcium phosphate and oyster shell (basically calcium carbonate). Current evidence suggests that most people absorb each of these equally well.

Look for the number of milligrams of calcium per tablet. Some supplements have relatively little calcium, making them an impractical source. Calcium carbonate has the highest concentration of calcium, followed by calcium phosphate, then calcium lactate. Consider the number of tablets you have to take to meet your daily quota. It's easier to take two or three than eight or ten.

Milk-Shunning Adults

Mom's no longer there to coax you to drain that glass, so perhaps milk's no longer on your menu, except in coffee or tea. For adults, and, for that matter, kids who won't drink milk, calcium intake is likely to be precariously low. Other food sources normally provide only 200 to 300 milligrams of calcium a day.

If milk just isn't your cup of tea, try disguising its taste, suggests Hausman. Use plenty of milk in pancakes, cereals, shakes and puddings. Add powdered milk to everything from creamy salad dressings to meat loaf. And make sure you're getting at least three servings a day of cheese, yogurt (try frozen soft-serve yogurt for a treat) or high-calcium nondairy foods, like sardines, oysters or shrimp.

If milk or other dairy products cause diarrhea and gas, you may be lactose intolerant. You lack an enzyme that allows your bowel to break down milk sugars. But that doesn't mean dairy products are entirely off-limits. Look for brands of milk in which the lactose has already been broken down, or add a powdered enzyme, available at drugstores, to your regular brand. Try yogurt, which has less lactose than milk, provided it has no added milk solids.

Some people with lactose intolerance can eat some dairy products without symptoms, and they usually have fewer symptoms if they mix dairy products with other foods. Lactose intolerance does not significantly impair your ability to absorb calcium.

Growing Teenagers

If you've got one, you know that teenagers are notorious for eating exactly what they want. And what they prefer usually comes in a bag from a drive-through window.

"Some fast foods can be good sources of calcium," says Ellen Coleman, R.D., of the Riverside Cardiac Fitness Center in Riverside, California. The average fast-food cheeseburger provides 150 milligrams of calcium; one-fourth of a 14-inch pizza, 290 milligrams; a taco with cheese, 110 milligrams; a ten-ounce vanilla shake, 325 milligrams.

Of course, these aren't foods you'd want to eat every day. "They have too much fat and too many calories for the amount of nutrients they deliver," Coleman says. She finds that most teenagers, when invited to indulge, also consume large quantities of calcium-rich chocolate milk, frozen yogurt, puddings, custards, cream soups, soufflés and cheese sauces.

The calcium RDA for ages 11 to 18 is 1,200 milligrams. That's as high as it is for pregnant women. And it's a level few teenagers seem to achieve. That concerns some bone-metabolism specialists, who say the best time to increase bone mass is before age 35. Scrimping on calcium during adolescence may be the perfect setup for osteoporosis later in life.

People with Low Stomach Acid

As they age, many people experience decreased stomach acidity. They probably won't have much trouble absorbing calcium from the foods they eat, since the food itself stimulates stomach acid production. But they may have problems taking in the calcium from supplements, especially on an empty stomach. Some acid is needed to absorb calcium carbonate, but an empty stomach usually contains none.

"It might be a good idea for older people and those with known impairment of gastric acid secretion to take their calcium supplement with meals," says Robert Recker, M.D., of the Creighton University School of Medicine, Omaha, Nebraska. Dr. Recker has found that the presence of a meal in the stomach is sufficient to permit normal absorption of calcium carbonate, even in patients with low stomach acid.

Or they might want to consider switching to calcium citrate, a water-soluble form of calcium. Dr. Recker found that when people with low stomach acid took their calcium without food, they absorbed only 5 percent of calcium carbonate. In contrast, they absorbed 45 percent of calcium citrate.

Kidney-Stone Formers

Almost everyone can safely consume up to 1,200 milligrams of calcium a day. "People who form kidney stones, though, shouldn't be taking calcium supplements without a doctor's supervision," says Charles Pak, M.D., chief of mineral metabolism at the University of Texas Health Science Center, Dallas. "In stone formers, calcium supplements lead to excessive calcium levels in the urine, which can aggravate stone formation."

Stone formers who want to take supplemental calcium might try calcium citrate, Dr. Pak says. This compound increases levels of urinary citrate, a substance that inhibits formation of calcium stones.

Pregnant and Lactating Women

Because estrogen levels are high during pregnancy, you have the potential for building bone tissue, provided you get plenty of calcium. Calcium demands are high during pregnancy — 1,200 milligrams a day. Most prenatal supplements don't provide much of the mineral, Coleman says. And obstetricians don't always pay calcium the attention it deserves. It may be up to you to beef up your diet to get enough, or to tell your doctor you want to take supplemental calcium. Calcium needs are even higher during breastfeeding than pregnancy, although the RDA is the same, Hausman says. "A woman who breastfeeds her baby for nine months loses three to four times as much calcium in her milk as she lost during her nine months of pregnancy."

Athletes

It's true that physical activity helps keep your bones strong. But exercise by itself is not enough. You need calcium, too.

And too much physical activity can actually hurt bones. Women runners who have stopped menstruating experience a rapid loss of calcium from the bones, probably because of a drop in estrogen levels. They need to train less and eat more, especially calcium-rich dairy foods.

Pectin's "One-Two" Punch for Better Health

Do you have high cholesterol? Diabetes? If you do, your bathroom cabinet probably contains medicines to control these problems. But maybe you should also be looking in the produce compartment of your refrigerator for help. You just might find it — in sweet oranges, crisp apples, crunchy carrots and tasty nuts and beans.

What's so special about these foods? They all contain a gelatinous fiber called pectin. It's the "glue" that holds together plant cells, and it is found in varying amounts in many fruits and vegetables. Home canners know pectin as a white powder, made from cull apples or grapefruit skin, that's used to firm up jellies. Producing perfect jam, though, is only a small act in pectin's repertoire of skills.

Researchers have found that pectin is one of the best substances there is for reducing high blood-cholesterol levels.

"As far as I can see, pectin is about the most effective fiber for reducing cholesterol levels," says Sheldon Reiser, Ph.D., director of the Carbohydrate Nutrition Laboratory at the U.S. Department of Agriculture's Human Nutrition Research Center in Beltsville, Maryland. Dr. Reiser recently completed a survey of pectin research.

"There have been a great number of studies, done with very diverse segments of the population, and they have confirmed pectin's role in reducing cholesterol levels," Dr. Reiser says. "The consistency of findings in these studies is very impressive."

Pectin Soaks Up Cholesterol

The studies show that pectin reduces blood levels of a harmful kind of cholesterol, known as LDL (low-density lipoprotein) cholesterol. It does this without also lowering levels of beneficial HDL (high-density lipoprotein) cholesterol. That is important because high levels of LDL cholesterol have been shown to multiply your risk of developing heart disease.

Pectin acts like a sponge in your intestines. It binds components of digestive fluids secreted by the liver and gallbladder. Some of these components, called bile salts, are formed from body stores of cholesterol. Normally, after the bile salts are used to digest food, they are reabsorbed into the body to be recycled. But when pectin combines with bile salts, the intestines can't reabsorb them, and they are excreted. That means the body has to dip into its cholesterol stores to make more bile salts. The more often it must do this, the lower its cholesterol stores, and the healthier your arteries. Studies have shown that pectin can absorb up to four times its weight in cholesterol.

Pectin seems to work best in people whose cholesterol levels are highest, Dr. Reiser says. It's particularly effective in people with a genetic tendency toward high cholesterol levels, reducing their blood levels by as much as 19 percent. In people with low to normal cholesterol levels, it has less effect.

How much pectin do you need to consume to see results? That depends, Dr. Reiser says. In most studies, pectin didn't begin to have a significant effect on cholesterol levels until people were getting 6 to 8 grams a day. Most studies found increasingly better results as more pectin was given, although most didn't use more than 15 grams a day.

"The trick is to find the lowest amount that works for you," Dr. Reiser says. You can do that by having a blood cholesterol test taken, then adding, say, 6 grams of pectin a day to your diet for a month, then having another blood test. Then, if you want, try adding another 2 to 4 grams of pectin, and in another month, have a second blood test. There's no good reason to overdo it, Dr. Reiser adds. "Once you get to a certain level of effectiveness, there's no indication that you can improve it by adding even more pectin, although there are enough studies where people have gotten 15 to 20 grams a day of pectin that indicate that it isn't harmful."

Vitamin C Boosts Effects

A few studies have noted that when extra vitamin C is added to your diet along with pectin, cholesterol levels drop even lower. Conveniently, some pectin-packed fruits and vegetables are also rich in vitamin C.

"The enzyme that starts converting cholesterol to bile acids is activated by vitamin C," Dr. Reiser explains. "With vitamin C you have the enzyme capability in your body to transform cholesterol into bile acids." People deficient in vitamin C produce less bile acid. If you're taking pectin, make sure you also get enough vitamin C. In one study, 15 grams of pectin and 450 milligrams of vitamin C daily were found to be very effective in reducing cholesterol levels.

Diabetics Can Benefit, Too

Pectin also works in ways that can help diabetics keep their blood sugar and insulin levels normal and stable. When it is consumed with a meal or in a glucose tolerance test, pectin reduces the subsequent rise in blood sugar and in insulin levels.

Pectin may work by slowing the absorption of sugar through the intestine. "It creates a kind of diffusion barrier on the intestinal lining," Dr. Reiser says. "It creates a thicker membrane barrier through which the glucose has to pass to be absorbed," so sugar is absorbed gradually, through a longer length of intestine.

In studies where pectin was effective in reducing blood sugar and insulin levels, people were getting from 10 to 14 grams with each meal.

Claims that pectin can help you lose weight without cutting calories haven't proved true, Dr. Reiser says. "To do that, it would have to cause malabsorption of food, and it doesn't do that," he says. In fact, unlike some other fibers, pectin seems not to interfere with vitamin or mineral absorption, which makes it safe even in large amounts.

Pectin May Help Bowel Disease

Studies done over a number of years have shown that pectin changes the structure of the cells lining the intestine. "In microscopic cross sections of intestinal lining, the villi [tiny, fingerlike projections that give the intestinal lining its velvety look] were taller in animals given pectin than in animals on the same diet without pectin," says John Rombeau, M.D., associate professor of surgery at the University of Pennsylvania Medical School, Philadelphia. Studies have confirmed that there is more intestinal cell turnover and growth in animals given pectin supplements.

In trying to see if these findings have any practical application, Dr. Rombeau decided to look at inflammatory bowel disease. He found that in rats with experimentally induced colitis, those that had pectin added to their diet healed much faster than those fed a fiber-free liquid diet. A study of the pectin-supplemented rats' intestinal cells showed more growth and bigger cells.

During a flare-up of colitis, standard medical treatment is to "rest" the bowel by stopping food and giving intravenous nourishment, Dr. Rombeau says. "Instead of doing that, we are trying to 'feed' the diseased intestine with a specific fuel that it might utilize."

In the colon, pectin is broken down into what are called short-chain fatty acids. The cells that line the colon can use these fatty acids directly as an energy source. "These fatty acids provide an important source of nourishment for these cells, helping them reproduce, grow and heal," Dr. Rombeau explains.

More research needs to be done before recommendations can be made, Dr. Rombeau notes. But he's hopeful pectin may soon play a role in the treatment of bowel disease. "It's inexpensive, harmless, and may have real potential for patients who need some intestinal healing," he says.

Researchers like Dr. Reiser feel pectin will work best as part of a well-balanced diet that includes plenty of fruits, vegetables, grains and beans.

"I think there is nothing to lose and everything to gain by eating pectin," Dr. Reiser says. "The foods containing pectin are good for you, and pectin has been shown to be effective. Once people begin to see clinical improvement, and feel better, they have the incentive to keep on this kind of dietary regimen."

Natural Healing Diets

Most of us, in one form or another, follow what we consider to be a prudent diet. We load up on grains, vegetables and fruits. We choose fish, chicken, low-fat dairy products and lean cuts of beef.

We eat this way because we know it's the only way to go if we expect to glide gracefully into old age.

But what if you're already sick? Are there diets that cure, not just prevent, disease? Doctors are finding that, in some cases, dietary changes are the only thing you need to do to stop, treat or control an illness. Most of these changes are modifications of the basic prudent diet we may have been following. More often than not, such healing diets have several points in common. Here are some eating programs that are proven healers.

The Elimination/Food Challenge Diet

Some people definitely know a food allergy when they meet one—hives or shortness of breath appear within minutes after they eat a food. But many sufferers may not be sure what foods are causing their congestion, stomach upsets, fatigue, headaches or skin rashes. That's where the elimination/food challenge diet comes in.

The premise of this diet is simple enough. First, stop eating all the foods you think might be causing your allergy symptoms. Then, when you are symptom free, add foods back one by one and note which cause symptoms to reappear.

There are several initial-phase allergy-free diets. Some doctors fast their patients on springwater for a few days. Others use a nonallergic, predigested liquid food. Most, though, put their patients on a limited diet of foods generally considered nonallergic, says Richard Podell, M.D., a New Providence, New Jersey, internist and allergist, and clinical associate professor at New Jersey's Robert Wood Johnson Medical School.

This diet may include lamb, rice, pears, springwater, salt, green beans, sweet potatoes and a cooking oil like pure safflower oil.

Dr. Podell keeps his patients on this diet for up to three weeks. "If they don't improve, food is probably not their problem," he says. "If they do improve, and many do, then we add new foods one at a time and see which trigger their symptoms."

Dr. Podell usually introduces each food back in three successive meals. "If they seem to react adversely, we put that food on our suspect list," he says. "We then go back and verify those foods with a second challenge."

People on this diet should make a point not to lose more than two pounds a week, Dr. Podell says. And they should be aware that a food-challenge response could be severe. Those with hives, general swelling, throat tightening, low blood pressure and asthma-type reactions should be challenged only under medical supervision.

The High Blood Pressure "Diet"

Just don't call it a diet, says Arlene Caggiula, R.D., Ph.D., associate professor of nutrition and epidemiology at the University of Pittsburgh School of Public Health. She prefers to call her long-term nondrug plan for reducing high blood pressure a "comprehensive eating program"—one that incorporates all dietary aspects of blood pressure control.

Reducing sodium intake to about two grams a day is an important aspect. "People can usually cut about two grams by not adding salt to foods," Dr. Caggiula says. They can eliminate two more grams by avoiding foods processed with sodium, such as ham, lunch meats and bacon. That leaves them with about two grams of sodium naturally occurring in foods. That's the only sodium she thinks people should eat.

Whittling weight down is her second recommendation. "Our program can easily be calorie-controlled to lose weight," Dr. Caggiula says. "You don't necessarily have to lose a lot of weight to see blood pressure drop. Most studies indicate that a 5 percent weight loss is enough for significant blood pressure lowering."

Limiting alcohol to no more than two drinks a day is important, Dr. Caggiula says.

"In large amounts, alcohol raises blood pressure," she says. "And people who are trying to lose weight shouldn't be wasting calories on alcohol. They need those calories for nutritious foods."

Cutting fat consumption is a crucial aspect of the program. "There's some thought that fats have their own independent effect on blood pressure," Dr. Caggiula says.

And blood pressure medications, especially diuretics, can raise levels of blood fats. "We want to make sure our eating program counteracts that effect," Dr. Caggiula says. She suggests cutting back to about 25 percent total fat, substituting fish and vegetable oils for red meat and butter, and limiting cholesterol intake to about 200 milligrams a day.

Foods rich in calcium and potassium are highlighted in this eating program. Those minerals work to control important functions of the vascular system. Adequate amounts may help keep blood pressure down. "We emphasize low-fat dairy products like skim milk and yogurt and high-potassium fruits and vegetables like bananas, apricots, raisins, cantaloupes, potatoes, dried beans and avocados," Dr. Caggiula says. "Potassium-rich foods also have a lot of other nutrients that could be helpful—vitamin A, beta-carotene, magnesium, vitamin C. When people choose these foods, they're maximizing their intake of many important nutrients."

The Diet for Irritable Bowel Syndrome

Doctors have discovered that the constipation and cramps of irritable bowel syndrome often can be eased with improved eating habits.

Adding more fiber may be all some people have to do, says Barbara Harland, R.D., Ph.D., associate professor, Department of Human Ecology, at Howard University, Washington, D.C. "Many of these people have been eating very little fiber," she says. "Simply increasing their intake to 25 to 30 grams of total dietary fiber a day regulates movement of food within the intestines and eliminates symptoms." Just switching to whole grain bread and cereals can make the difference.

In some sensitive people, milk and dairy products, colas, chocolate, corn, eggs, soybeans and peanuts, citrus fruits, tomatoes, wheat, cinnamon, pork, beef, onions or garlic may irritate the gastrointestinal tract, producing diarrhea and cramping. Limiting the amount that you eat of those foods often provides relief, Dr. Harland says.

The Low, Low Fat, Heart Disease Diet

The American Heart Association (AHA) now recommends a diet of no more than 30 percent fat to prevent heart disease. That's about 10 percent less than the normal American diet contains. The Pritikin diet, on the other hand, cuts fats way back to about 10 percent of total calories.

"I think the AHA is compromising. They're trying to make recommendations they think are realistic, but which certainly aren't optimum in terms of preventing heart disease," says Jay Kenney, R.D., Ph.D., nutrition educator for the Pritikin Longevity Center, Santa Monica, California. "The AHA's concern about the Pritikin diet is not that it won't work; it's that it's unrealistic, that no one will follow it."

Certainly, not everyone can stick to the austere food plan, but many of the highly motivated people who come to the Pritikin Center for training successfully revise their eating habits rather than suffer chest pain, fatigue and the side effects of heavy-duty drugs.

The Pritikin plan offers both "regression" and maintenance diets. Both aim for about 10 percent of total calories from fat. The regression (or therapeutic) diet limits daily cholesterol intake to no more than 25 milligrams; the maintenance diet allows more animal protein and may have up to 100 milligrams of cholesterol per day. Both diets are very satisfying and high in fiber (40 to 60 grams a day).

Both emphasize whole grains, beans, vegetables, nonfat dairy products and fruit. The regression diet allows 3½ ounces of fish, chicken or lean meat a week. The maintenance diet allows up to 3½ ounces of meat, fish or poultry per day. Sodium is restricted to less than two grams a day.

Both diets completely eliminate refined sugar, egg yolks, butter, all refined fats and oils, whole milk, cheeses made from whole milk, organ meats, oils, nuts, seeds and caffeine.

"The benefit of the diet is in direct proportion to how closely you follow it and how low you can get your blood cholesterol levels," Dr. Kenney says. "If you can get your cholesterol below 160, evidence is quite good that you get at least some reversal of atherosclerosis."

He does caution that long-affected vessels have some irreversible scarring and calcification. "But cholesterol deposits and dead and dying tissue are taken out of those lesions when you're on a very low-fat diet," he says. "Even older lesions can be shrunk up to 50 percent, and early lesions—fatty streaks—have proved to be 100 percent reversible in animal research."

Medical experts who disagree that a low-fat diet can reverse heart disease still readily acknowledge that the diet can alleviate many symptoms. By making blood cells less likely to clump together, especially in small blood vessels, a low-fat diet really cuts down on angina pain. And it makes a heart attack much less likely to occur.

The "No More Kidney Stones" Diet

Dietary changes help many people with kidney stones, says Steven Kanig, M.D., director of nephrology for the Lovelace Medical Center, Albuquerque, New Mexico, and clinical assistant professor of medicine at the University of New Mexico. But analysis of the mineral content of urine, blood and kidney stones is needed to determine exactly what dietary changes will work for each individual.

One recommendation that does seem to work for many is drinking more water, from three to four quarts a day—sometimes even more if you sweat a lot—to increase urine output to about two quarts a day.

"This decreases the concentration of minerals in the urine, making it less likely for minerals to precipitate out as stones," Dr. Kanig says. One study found that this simple measure cut repeat occurrences of stones in 60 percent of the patients involved.

Eating less protein may also help some kidney-stone formers, Dr. Kanig says. Too much protein may lead to higher than normal levels of uric acid in the urine, which can cause tiny crystals to form in the kidneys. These provide the nucleus for several kinds of kidney stones. Most people could easily cut their total protein intake by a third or more.

Reducing salt is also recommended, especially for people who have some kidney damage, Dr. Kanig says. "In people with kidney insufficiency, a sudden increase in salt could mean a rapid rise in blood pressure due to fluid retention." In kidney-stone formers, a high salt intake can cause increased concentrations of other minerals, like calcium, in the urine. That's something they want to avoid.

"I simply tell people not to add salt at the table and to avoid foods that are obviously salty," Dr. Kanig says. "That seems to work pretty well."

Most people form stones made of a combination of calcium and oxalate, a chemical found in spinach and some other green leafy vegetables, tea and chocolate. Some, but not all, people benefit from restricting their intake of calcium- and oxalate-containing foods.

"I'd tell people who are eating huge amounts of these foods to cut back," Dr. Kanig says. He also advises kidney-stone formers who are taking extra calcium, or any other vitamin or mineral, to talk with their doctor.

"Unfortunately, for many people who have had multiple kidney stones, medications are also necessary to significantly decrease new stone formation," says Dr. Kanig. "However, the dietary measures discussed make the overall treatment program much more successful."

Don't Let Anemia Drain Your Vigor

"I feel so much better—I never realized I haven't had the energy I should."

This is a common reaction from people who've bounced back from iron-deficiency anemia, a common blood disorder whose hallmark sign is feeling tired and washed-out.

"Very often we'll give an iron supplement to people who are only slightly anemic, and they'll report feeling more energetic," says Suzanne McClure, M.D., assistant professor of medicine in the Division of Hematology-Oncology at the University of Texas Medical Branch in Galveston.

"We have seen reports," adds Annette Natow, R.D., Ph.D., professor of nutrition at Adelphi University in Garden City, New York, "showing that just having low iron intake—without being full-blown anemic—might result in some people having concentration ability and immune system responses that aren't up to par."

It's no wonder then, that people who develop more pronounced iron deficiency may have fatigue compounded by depression, fainting spells, headaches, heartburn, irritability, itching, pale lips and skin, poor appetite or memory, a sore tongue or brittle nails. Also, people with angina may notice their condition getting worse.

Supply and Demand

The body's energy levels are taxed when it doesn't get enough iron for one of the mineral's chief functions: producing hemoglobin. It's iron-based hemoglobin that carries oxygen to tissues and cells to energize them. If iron levels drop, then hemoglobin and energy fade, too.

Doctors first look at what factors in a person's lifestyle might be acting alone or in combination to deplete iron stores.

Iron deficiency and anemia often hit people who've set themselves up this way: Neglecting to put enough iron-rich foods in their diet, they don't have enough of the mineral packed away in their bone marrow for "emergencies," as they should. Then they start to lose blood for expected reasons (menstruation, pregnancy) or unexpected reasons (ulcers, hemorrhoids). The blood loss bills the body for extra iron to make up for what's lost, and the body can't pay the balance.

That is just one anemia scenario. Prolonged, paltry iron intake alone, without a blood loss condition, can make some people anemic. On the other hand, it's possible to not get enough iron and escape any adverse effects.

A doctor can do a full-scale blood chemistry test to analyze several factors, one being hemoglobin levels, and determine if iron is in short supply. He or she also checks to see if any of the following risk factors are coming into play.

If You're a Menstruating Woman, You're the Most Likely Candidate for Anemia ● "It's impossible for most women to get anywhere near the iron they need from their diets," says Dr. Natow. "If a woman's on a 1,000-calorie reducing diet, for example, she's probably only taking in 6 milligrams of iron—pitifully less than the Recommended Dietary Allowance [RDA] of 18 milligrams. Even if she eats 2,000 calories a day, which is generally way more than figure-conscious women allow themselves, her iron intake will average only about 12 milligrams. Add to that the fact that most women choose iron-poor 'diet foods,' such as cottage cheese, yogurt, lettuce and fruit juice, for a good percentage of what calories they will consume, and iron deficiency becomes even more likely."

Menstruation compounds the iron problem even more. Women with heavier flows face greater odds of being iron deficient; users of birth control pills enjoy a lessened risk usually due to lighter periods. Pregnancy especially takes its toll on iron by assigning the mother's iron supply to double-duty nourishing.

"A woman can suffer from somewhat of an iron deficit after years of simply being female," Dr. McClure notes. She once attended a health fair for hospital employees where all female nurses had their iron levels evaluated. "Over one-quarter of the women were iron deficient, and a few were outright anemic. These were health-conscious people who knew all about, and cared about, eating well, but menstrual blood loss was still sapping their iron. This is why women should have their blood checked at regular intervals," says Dr. McClure.

Gastrointestinal Disorders May Contribute to Anemia ● This is the main factor that puts a man at risk for iron-deficiency anemia, because men easily consume their RDA of ten milligrams of iron each day.

Many things might cause gastrointestinal bleeding. Some, like hemorrhoids, can obviously be noticed by a person. Other conditions may go undetected without an internal exam—benign or malignant polyps, or bleeding ulcers, for example. Irritable bowel syndrome can sometimes cause blood loss, too. "When you hit 40 and older, you enter a higher risk group for GI conditions," Dr. McClure explains. "You can't always notice blood in your stool, either, because it may not be red. It's a good idea to do one of the home stool tests, or get one from your doctor, every year. This isn't on people's list of top ten things to do, but it's an important diagnostic test that shouldn't be avoided." The American Cancer Society's guidelines of having a thorough colon and rectal exam between ages 40 and 50, followed by another exam every three to five years, are also wise measures.

One additional stomach irritant is aspirin. It can cause bleeding in people who take large amounts (it's not uncommon for arthritis sufferers to take four tablets every four hours to relieve pain, says Dr. Natow).

Children Have an Increased Need for Iron ● "A growing child needs to get lots of iron to handle the job of building all the new red blood cells in the growing volume of blood," explains Myron Winick, M.D., a New York City pediatrician and director of the Institute of Human Nutrition at Columbia University College of Physicians and Surgeons. "His or her diet needs lots of iron-rich meats and vegetables or iron-fortified cereals. If the child's a picky eater, iron supplements are in order to make sure the body can keep up with the increased iron need.

"Babies, until about their first birthday, should either keep receiving breast milk or iron-fortified formula," stresses Dr. Winick. "Starting a baby on whole milk earlier than this deprives him or her of iron, not only because whole milk simply doesn't have any, but also because it contains high amounts of protein, which can cause microscopic bleeding in the gastrointestinal tract and cause blood to be lost in the stool. Breast milk's iron is very well absorbed, on the other hand."

Certain Dietary Factors Inhibit Iron Absorption ● Coffee and tea contain tannin, a substance that, if the beverages are taken with meals, can cut the amount of iron absorbed by 40 to 95 percent. If these drinks are one of your favorite pleasures, try waiting until an hour or two after a meal to have them.

Iron is also blocked by the phosphates in ice cream, candy bars, baked goods, beer and soft drinks. EDTA, an additive in many canned and processed foods, has the same inhibiting trait. (Check labels for EDTA if you're concerned.) Calcium, important for bones though it may be, may also be guilty of iron inhibition when it's taken as a supplement with meals. Bess D. Hughes, M.D., of the U.S. Department of Agriculture's Human Nutrition Research Center on Aging at Tufts University in Boston, notes that women seeking to guard against osteoporosis should take their calcium supplements on an empty stomach so as not to interfere with iron absorption.

Gatekeepers of Iron

In addition of being aware of iron sappers, you can make the most of iron enhancers.

Beef, veal, fish, lamb, poultry and game multiply iron absorption fourfold. These meats encourage your body to take in nonheme iron, a form of the mineral that isn't easy to absorb.

Vitamin C lends a hand in nonheme iron absorption, too. Dr. Natow suggests that if you take an iron supplement, you drink vitamin C-rich orange juice at the same time. Good vitamin C bets are citrus fruits, cabbage, peppers, tomatoes, broccoli, cantaloupe and strawberries.

Another iron-boosting benefit from vegetables and citrus fruits is that they contain lots of folate, a B vitamin that iron needs to pair up with for optimal performance. Folate's also abundant in liver, beans and seafood.

The iron-pot trick can boost iron intake threefold. As your food simmers in the skillet, some of the pot's iron comes off into the food and strengthens nutritional value.

Finally, the following foods, and perhaps an iron supplement if needed, are the best at keeping your iron stores stocked.

● Beef liver, roast beef, lean ground beef, white meat chicken, dark meat turkey.
● Prunes, dried apricots, raisins, blackstrap molasses, sunflower seeds.
● Lima beans, soybeans, broccoli, spinach, peas, beet greens, kidney beans, endive, escarole.

Nutrition for Your Innermost Youth

Deepening wrinkles or the gray hairs that almost seem to pop up overnight may be more visible signs of aging. But the aging that goes on *inside* our bodies actually has more far-reaching consequences.

Much of the internal damage that accumulates over a lifetime, and the diseases that go with it, may be linked to mischievous molecules inside us called free radicals, says Sheldon Hendler, M.D., Ph.D., author of *The Complete Guide to Anti-Aging Nutrients*. But we don't have to accept passively what the years dish out. "Free radicals are something we can identify, measure and do battle with."

Free radicals are as wild as their name, says Dr. Hendler. "But actually, they don't like being 'free,' at least in the sense of remaining single or unattached."

They are typically substances with unpaired electrons, and that puts them in a "desperate tizzy to get hitched to almost anything they can grab onto" that will pair up their missing electrons. When they latch onto something, it's known as oxidation. And oxidation can "rust" the body almost as it does metal.

This oxidation occurs most readily in fats. So cell membranes, which are rich in fat molecules, are prime targets. A free-radical attack on the cells could kill or severely damage them—leaving them vulnerable to cancer or other diseases.

"Given the fact that fats account for more than 40 percent of the total calories in the typical American diet, it is not difficult to see how we might be exposed to . . . extensive free-radical activity," says Dr. Hendler.

Free radicals, which are created by the body's normal metabolism, as well as by radiation, ozone exposure and cancer-causing chemicals, do have a purpose, however. Some play a role in the body's enzyme reactions and help kill invading bacteria. But the extras are bad guys. They leave not only destruction in their path but also their imprint, a pigment called lipofuscin, which causes age spots.

59

The Free-Radical Diseases

"The details of how free radicals cause disease are really not fully known, but they do," says Denham Harman, M.D., Ph.D., of the University of Nebraska College of Medicine, Omaha. "There is a great deal of data indicating that, when all is said and done, free radicals are the major cause of many diseases."

So far free radicals have been implicated in a long list of problems that accompany aging, including cancer, atherosclerosis, high blood pressure, Alzheimer's disease, osteoarthritis and immune deficiency, says Dr. Harman.

But there is good news. Substances called antioxidants can neutralize free radicals by pairing up their electrons. Vitamins C and E and the mineral selenium are known to be antioxidants that, along with antioxidant enzymes produced by the body, help to protect the body's cells.

Researchers at the Institute of Food and Nutrition in Warsaw, Poland, found that vitamins E and C can decrease the level of free radicals in the blood. One hundred people aged 60 to 100 were given either vitamin E (approximately 200 international units) or vitamin C (400 milligrams) or both every day for a year. The vitamin E alone decreased the free radical level by 26 percent. The vitamin C decreased it by 13 percent. And the group taking both E and C decreased their levels by 25 percent.

Other researchers are finding evidence that dietary antioxidants are able to prevent free radical activity and some of its unpleasant side effects throughout the body. Here are some recent findings.

Cataracts ● Vitamin C may protect the lenses of the eyes from the constant bombardment and damage by light and oxygen that makes them vulnerable to cataracts.

"We fed guinea pigs vitamin C in both high and low doses and found that with high doses you get three to five times as much vitamin C in the lens," says Allen Taylor, Ph.D., director of the Laboratory for Nutrition and Cataract Research at the U.S. Department of Agriculture's (USDA) Human Nutrition Research Center on Aging at Tufts University in Boston.

"We took those lenses and artificially aged them by exposing them to ultraviolet light in the exact same wavelengths and
similar doses that people encounter in a normal day. We
showed that the lenses with more vitamin C were better able to
withstand the photo-oxidative stress that we used to artificially
age them.

"To our minds, this suggests that vitamin C may be very
important in delaying the onset of damage to proteins in the
lens of the eye. Such changes are associated with cataract
formation," says Dr. Taylor.

Respiratory Diseases ● "Ozone is one of the strongest oxidants known, so it has the potential for doing tremendous
damage to the lungs and to the entire body when you breathe it
in smoggy air," says William A. Pryor, Ph.D., director of the
Biodynamics Institute at Louisiana State University, Baton
Rouge. "And every major city in the United States is exceeding
the Clean Air Act's standard for recommended levels of ozone."

Ozone weakens the body's ability to use oxygen for energy.
The effects can be subtle or they can kill. "Deaths in nursing
homes, for example, sharply increase on smog-alert days in the
Los Angeles basin," says Dr. Pryor. "On high smog-alert days,
there's high ozone, which causes decreased lung function.
And that increases stress on the elderly." There is also increasing evidence that ozone, like some other oxidants, may cause
cancer, says Dr. Pryor.

Numerous studies have shown that susceptibility to lung
damage from ozone can be reduced by adding vitamin E
supplements to animals' diets, says Dr. Pryor. "And animals
given vitamin E live appreciably longer than vitamin E-deficient
animals when exposed to ozone."

Cancer ● Vitamins A, E and C and selenium may play roles
in preventing some cancers, says Ronald Ross Watson, Ph.D.,
of the Department of Family and Community Medicine at
Arizona Health Sciences Center in Tucson. Studies have concluded that:

● Areas with low selenium content in the soil and water have
more deaths from cancers of the esophagus, stomach and

rectum. The formation in the body of the antioxidant enzyme glutathione peroxidase depends on selenium. Selenium may also enhance immunity, inhibiting cancer.

● Vitamin A deficiency may increase the risk of cancers of the lung, larynx, bladder, esophagus, stomach, colon, rectum and prostate.

● Vitamin C reduces the risk of cervical dysplasia, a precancerous condition.

● Vitamin E may have a role in reducing the risk of lung cancer. Researchers at the Johns Hopkins School of Hygiene and Public Health in Baltimore found that those who had the lowest levels of the vitamin in their blood had a 2½ times higher risk of lung cancer than people with the highest levels.

Senility ● "It hasn't been proved, but many people have suggested that senile dementia has its origin in free-radical damage," says Jeffrey Blumberg, Ph.D., of the USDA Human Nutrition Research Center on Aging at Tufts. "We don't know how free-radical damage might cause senile dementia, but one way it could do that is by damaging nerves in the brain.

"We have shown in our study that free-radical damage occurred in the brain more readily in old animals than in young animals. We also found that vitamin E protects against that damage. When we gave the animals vitamin E-deficient diets, the damage was much greater. The effects were similar in the liver, but we were mainly interested in looking at the brain."

Immune Deficiency ● "We know that immune function declines with age," says Dr. Blumberg. "And we've found in our animal studies that high levels of vitamin E are capable of reversing this decline. Not totally reversing to levels comparable to those in younger animals, but partially."

Our immune systems play an important role in resisting diseases, including cancer. "If the immune system is less vigorous, then disease has a much greater chance of winning," says Dr. Blumberg.

How to Fight Free Radicals

It is reasonable to expect that we can stay healthier and live longer, increasing average life expectancy (now 74.8 years)

HOW TO GET ANTIOXIDANTS INTO YOUR DIET

Research has shown that antioxidants often help each other out, having even more power together than they have alone. So including in your diet the foods listed below might help boost your body's fight against free radicals.

Outstanding food sources of vitamin A include:

Broccoli	Spinach
Cantaloupe	Sweet potatoes
Carrots	

The best food sources of vitamin C include:

Broccoli	Green peppers
Brussels sprouts	Orange juice
Cantaloupe	Oranges
Grapefruit juice	Papayas

The best food sources of vitamin E include:

Almonds	Sunflower seed oil
Hazelnuts	Sunflower seeds
Pecans	Wheat germ oil
Raw wheat germ	

The best food sources of selenium include:

Broccoli	Seafood
Cabbage	Whole grain cereal and bread
Onions	

The amounts of selenium in foods may vary according to the levels of the mineral in the soils where they were produced. In general, soils in the West contain more selenium than those in the East.

5 or more years while possibly increasing the maximum life span slightly beyond 100 years, says Dr. Harman.

The probability of developing any one of the "free radical diseases" may be decreased by eating a diet rich in natural antioxidants, such as vitamins E and C, and low in total fat (including unsaturated fats), and by not overeating, says Dr. Harman. Free radicals are by-products of our metabolism. The more you eat, the more free radicals your body creates and has to contend with, he says.

By doing all you can to put the lid on free radicals, you'll be helping to preserve your youthfulness where it really counts—inside.

Nutrition Supplement Updates

How to Squeeze the Most Goodness Out of Your Food and Supplements

If you eat three square meals a day or take vitamin supplements, you might think you're getting adequate nutrition. You could be wrong.

Nutrition isn't that simple or direct. Your body doesn't always make the best use of all the vitamins you take in, either in food or in supplements. Some vitamins never get to where they can do the most good; others sail through your system without being absorbed.

The same is true of minerals. In fact, when it comes to figuring out how to make the most of your vitamins, minerals are often part of the plan.

If you want to squeeze every available microgram from your vitamins and minerals, it helps to understand some of the ways in which nutrients help each other along.

Here are some tips to help you make the most of your nutrients.

Eat Small, Nutritious Meals and Snacks ● All the nutrients your body takes in at a big meal can be hard to swallow, says John Pinto, Ph.D., assistant professor of nutrition and medicine at Cornell University Medical College and assistant member at Memorial Sloan-Kettering Cancer Center.

"If you stop and think how some people eat a large amount of protein and carbohydrates at one meal, they really swamp their system with this influx of nutrients all at one time," Dr. Pinto says. "And many of those nutrients won't be absorbed. That's because it's easier for the gastrointestinal tract to absorb nutrients from small amounts of food over a small period of time."

If you want to squeeze more nutritional value from your diet, scale down your main meals and eat healthful snacks— like a piece of fruit, crisp raw vegetables, a whole grain muffin or a glass of milk—in between. You'll give your body a chance to absorb nutrients most efficiently, says Dr. Pinto.

Take Your Vitamin C in Small, Divided Doses ● "The higher you dose at a single time, the smaller percentage of vitamin C you absorb," explains Mark Levine, M.D., a researcher at the National Institutes of Health in Bethesda, Maryland. "If you take 100 milligrams at one time, you get something like 90 percent absorption. If you go up to a gram [1,000 milligrams], it's approximately 50 percent absorption, and so on."

Instead of taking one large tablet of vitamin C, then, divide the same amount into smaller doses to be taken throughout the day.

"Let's say you choose to take two grams [2,000 milligrams] of vitamin C," says Dr. Levine. "You would increase the percentage of absorption if you took 500 milligrams four times a day, or 1,000 milligrams twice a day, instead of taking it all at once."

For Better Iron Absorption, Get More Vitamin C ● "Vitamin C enhances absorption of other nutrients, particularly iron," says Dr. Levine.

When we talk about iron, most of us think of foods like beef, poultry, fish and eggs. But not all iron is the same. Only about 10 percent of the iron in vegetables and grains—called nonheme (nonblood) iron—is absorbed. In contrast, we absorb from 15 to 30 percent of the iron found in meats, which is called heme iron.

Vitamin C is what is known as an iron enhancer. It helps convert the nonheme iron into a form the body can absorb.

If you want to make the most of your iron, eat more foods that are rich in vitamin C along with iron-rich foods, like lean meat, fish, poultry, leafy green vegetables and whole grains.

One way to improve the absorption of the iron in your beans and vegetables might be to add a thick, spicy tomato sauce. A piece of fruit for dessert, instead of that slab of double-fudge cake you've been coveting, is a healthier alternative if you want to boost your absorption of iron from your meal. If you take an iron supplement, wash it down with a little orange juice.

Take Fat-Soluble Vitamins with Foods Containing Fat ● Vitamins A, D and E are absorbed in the intestine in the presence of fat. Consequently, if you take fat-soluble vitamins on an empty stomach, you might flush out most of the vitamins before they can be absorbed.

"It's reasonable to take fat-soluble vitamins with foods that contain a small amount of fat—for example, a glass of low-fat [1 or 2 percent] milk," says Cedric Garland, Dr.P.H., professor of community and family medicine at the University of California at San Diego. "A moderate amount of fat would cause the secretion of digestive enzymes that work on fats, which should enhance absorption of the fat-soluble vitamins. Without a small amount of fat, a portion of those vitamins washes right through the intestine without being absorbed."

What about those of us on a low-fat diet? Don't worry, says Dr. Garland. "From a practical point of view, a diet containing 15 to 20 percent fat would still be sufficient to absorb fat-soluble vitamins."

To Move Calcium Along, Get Enough Vitamin D ● You can take calcium supplements every day and still leave your bones and teeth crying out for more . . . if you don't get enough vitamin D along with the mineral. Without vitamin D, calcium is not absorbed.

If you want to make sure you're getting enough of both nutrients, says Dr. Garland, one convenient way to do so is to drink milk, which contains plenty of calcium and vitamin D.

But drinking milk is only one way to boost your vitamin D. Perhaps the easiest way for most of us to make sure we get enough vitamin D is to take a stroll in the sunlight. Your skin manufactures vitamin D on its own, but it needs ultraviolet rays from sunlight to start the wheels turning.

How much sun to you need to make vitamin D? "Just 15 minutes a day, with sunlight on your hands and face, should be enough in most cases," says Dr. Garland. The walk will do you good, too, since weight-bearing exercise enhances the movement of calcium to your bones.

Take Your Calcium with Food ● Not all of us consume enough dairy products to keep us in calcium balance. Among healthy adults, pregnant and lactating women need the most. The RDA for this group is 1,200 milligrams of calcium daily. To get this amount of calcium, you would have to drink four to five glasses of milk a day. People who are at risk for osteoporosis may need even more, though the precise amount hasn't been firmly established.

If you don't get enough dietary calcium, you might take a supplement. But merely taking a supplement doesn't guarantee you the best results. Some calcium supplements are absorbed best in an acid environment. This is especially a problem for many people over the age of 60, whose production of stomach acid may be lower.

The solution is to take your calcium with a meal. This will stimulate your stomach to produce enough acid.

Food also helps improve the absorption of other nutrients. "It's best that nutrients be consumed with a meal," says Dr. Pinto. "The very sight of food begins to stimulate the appetite, triggering the release of various enzymes. Also, hormonal responses begin to register. With food in the mouth, insulin rises. Intestinal blood flow increases, preparing to help transport food through the body and move nutrients from the intestine into the bloodstream."

Take Your Calcium Supplements at Bedtime ● Timing of the dose could improve your body's absorption of the mineral, too. Morris Notelovitz, M.D., a gynecologist from the University of Florida at Gainesville, has suggested taking calcium supplements just before you turn in.

During the day, your body gets the calcium it needs from food. At night, when no food is coming in, your body still needs to maintain normal blood levels of calcium, so it raids the only source available to it—your skeleton.

A calcium supplement just before bed should keep your blood levels near normal and protect your bones from this nightly invasion. But if you have low stomach acid, remember the previous tip and swallow the calcium with a glass of low-fat milk to stimulate the production of stomach acids.

Keep Your Vitamins in the Safety Zone

To most of us, vitamins are as harmless as a kiss on the cheek. They are those tiny tablets or capsules that we take regularly to compensate for what may be lacking in an unbalanced diet. And even if we take a few extra milligrams here and there in the hope of dealing with or preventing health problems, the doses are usually sensible and safe.

Things can get a bit out of hand, however. After a report in the morning newspaper that vitamin X may prevent cancer, or a spot on the evening news that a certain mineral may help you live to be 100, some people are tempted to add larger doses to their daily routine.

The problem comes as the doses start to inch upward. Without realizing it, you could unintentionally be close to a megadose level, which should be taken only under a physician's direction. There's increasing evidence that too much of some nutrients may be harmful. The fat-soluble vitamins that can accumulate in the body, such as vitamins A and D, are particularly suspect.

Your goal is to stay within the vitamin safety zone, that range beginning at the U.S. Recommended Daily Allowance (USRDA) and ending "at the level that is still safe and well below the toxicity level," says John Hathcock, Ph.D., a vitamin toxicity expert with the U.S. Food and Drug Administration's (FDA) experimental nutritional section.

It's not easy for a vitamin-consuming public to decide where to draw the line between safe and excessive micrograms, milligrams or international units. "There are no officially established limits for maximum doses. We've spent a lot of time debating and establishing the USRDAs at the low end, but no one's set suggested guidelines for the other end," says Dr. Hathcock.

The simplest solution is to rely on food for most of your essential nutrients. "Nature has helped us out tremendously by giving our bodies the ability to get almost all the necessary vitamins and minerals we need from logical food consumption," says nutrition researcher Virginia Vivian, Ph.D., of Ohio State University. "Granted, you may need extra amounts of some nutrients, but a multiple vitamin will usually do."

That's easier said than done, however. Research has shown that many people either don't eat enough or do not eat balanced meals. Then there are people with medical conditions, pregnant women, the elderly and others who may have increased needs for specific nutrients.

That is why so many people turn to supplements. An FDA survey shows that about 40 percent of the general population takes supplements daily, with women taking more than men. Among the elderly, surveys show that between 66 and 72 percent take supplements.

It's also estimated that 5 to 10 percent of the people who take supplements ingest megadoses, defined by some researchers as ten times the USRDA or more, of certain vitamins and minerals. In light of this, some nutrition experts have stopped trying to tell people that they don't need vitamins, and instead have started advising them how to supplement wisely.

If you're wondering whether your own personal vitamin program falls within safe bounds, the answer's not easily had. "There are no reference guides or tables you can check to see what levels of vitamins trigger harmful effects," says Paul Saltman, Ph.D., a professor of biology doing research in nutrition at the University of California at San Diego. "That's because the danger levels vary from person to person and depend on factors such as weight, health status, metabolism, diet, nutritional status, the form of the nutrient and how often you take it. The safest approach is to accept the fact that there is no scientific evidence that massive doses have any benefits."

The Safety Zones

You may wish to check the following list of the more common vitamins and minerals to see where your dosages fit in. The "maximum" levels are approximately compiled from discussions with experts and surveys of the latest available data. These numbers should be viewed as general guidelines only, intended to help you make sure you're safe. This does not necessarily mean that it's appropriate or advisable to increase your intake to these limits. Also keep in mind that all metabolisms are not created equal. Although the most current information may suggest that a vitamin is relatively harmless, some people with unusual metabolic traits may react adversely to even the safest nutrient.

When considering your current total intake, don't neglect to add in the amounts in your multiple, if you take one each day. In other words, if you're taking a vitamin A supplement, don't think that's all the A you're getting. It's probably in your multiple, also.

Vitamin A ● Scientists have a keen new interest in this fat-soluble vitamin because of its link to cancer prevention. It speeds healing, aids vision and fights infection and skin diseases. Vitamin A is also highly toxic in large doses because it accumulates in organ tissues, primarily the liver. Headaches, blurred vision, nausea, hair loss, itchy eyes, aching bones or skin sores are signs that you may be taking too much. *USRDA:* 5,000 international units. *Maximum:* 25,000 international units.

(Beta-carotene, a carotenoid that offers many of the same benefits as vitamin A, appears to be safer than A in large doses. "So far, it looks relatively harmless, and you should consider taking it instead of the riskier vitamin A," says Dr. Saltman. Be aware, however, that large doses of vitamin E can interfere with beta-carotene absorption.)

Thiamine (B₁) and Riboflavin (B₂) ● There are very few reports of people experiencing adverse effects from either of these two B vitamins, partly because there's little if any evidence that large doses offer health benefits. *USRDA for thiamine:* 1.5 milligrams; *USRDA for riboflavin:* 1.7 milligrams. *Maximum for each:* 25 milligrams.

Niacin ● Studies have shown that this B vitamin may play a role in lowering cholesterol and triglyceride levels. But some people who take large doses in the form of nicotinic acid may experience niacin flush—a burning, itching, tingling sensation usually in the face, neck, arms and upper chest that may persist for half an hour or longer. Doses large enough to trigger this reaction may also cause reddening of the skin, nausea, headaches, cramps, diarrhea and feelings of faintness. *USRDA:* 20 milligrams. *Maximum:* 50 milligrams.

Vitamin B$_6$ (pyridoxine) ● Many women went running for this member of the B-complex family after reports that it helps ease premenstrual stress symptoms. "More research is needed to confirm that claim, but we have established that large doses can cause nerve damage," says Dr. Saltman. Numbness of the feet or hands may be a sign to reduce your intake. *USRDA:* 2 milligrams. *Maximum:* 50 milligrams.

Vitamin B$_{12}$ ● Although vitamin B$_{12}$ is vital to healthy blood and a normal nervous system, there's little scientific evidence that massive doses will either harm or help. *USRDA:* 6 micrograms. *Maximum:* 25 micrograms.

Pantothenate ● There is no known toxicity level, but caution should still be exercised since "we're just beginning to explore the effects of megadoses of some of these vitamins," says Dr. Saltman. *USRDA:* 10 milligrams. *Maximum:* 50 milligrams.

Vitamin C (ascorbic acid) ● Surveys continue to show that vitamin C is the most popular vitamin supplement, dominating the nutritional supermarket for the past decade. Scientific findings suggesting that it helps fight cancer, boosts immunity against colds and infections, speeds healing of wounds and aids in combating cardiovascular disease have made it one of the most megadosed vitamins. Although it's water soluble and excesses are usually excreted, large doses have been known to cause diarrhea and abdominal cramps in some people. Too much vitamin C may also interfere with certain medical tests, such as checking sugar levels in diabetics, or looking for blood in stools. *USRDA:* 60 milligrams. *Maximum:* 500 to 1,000 milligrams.

(The need for ascorbic acid varies considerably from one person to the next. Exposure to illness, tobacco smoke, pollutants, certain drugs, burns, trauma, surgery, alcohol and other stressors may increase the need. So may pregnancy and aging. Some nutritional researchers now regard the USRDA as too low for optimal health.)

Vitamin D ● Another fat-soluble vitamin that can accumulate in your body, vitamin D is usually obtained from sunshine. It's a crucial link in the process that helps calcium strengthen bones, and it is essential for women in their osteoporosis-prone years. People who live in regions where winters are long and exposure to sunlight is infrequent may need to take supplemental vitamin D. Muscle weakness, joint pain, headaches, nausea and vomiting may be signs that you should reduce your dosage. *USRDA:* 400 international units. *Maximum:* 400 international units.

(If you drink a quart of vitamin D-enriched milk daily, or get out in the sun year-round, you may not need D supplementation.)

Vitamin E ● Many people take vitamin E for its possible usefulness as an antioxidant, preventing premature aging or damage to body cells. "But in excessively large doses, vitamin E can upset the balance of other fat-soluble vitamins, and it can interfere with the function of vitamins A and K," says Dr. Vivian. Nausea, gastric problems or muscle weakness may be signs of too much. *USRDA:* 30 international units. *Maximum:* 600 international units.

Calcium ● More and more scientific investigations are suggesting that calcium helps prevent and treat the weakened, brittle bones that characterize osteoporosis. It also appears that postmenopausal women need more than the USRDA because their bodies' natural calcium-absorbing abilities decrease with age. Large doses may cause kidney stones in people prone to stone formation. *USRDA:* 1,000 milligrams. *Maximum:* 1,500 milligrams.

Chromium and Selenium ● The USRDAs for these two trace minerals have yet to be set. *Suggested range for each:* 50 to 200 micrograms. *Maximum for each:* 100 micrograms. (This assumes a dietary intake of 100 micrograms.)

Iron ● This mineral is enormously important to human health, preventing and curing iron-deficiency anemia. Iron supplements are widely used in the United States, but reports of iron overload are rare. In those cases where too much is taken, nausea, abdominal cramping, constipation and diarrhea can result. *USRDA:* 18 milligrams. *Maximum:* 30 milligrams.

(Needs for supplemental iron will vary. Vegetarians, women who are on low-calorie diets or are pregnant or nursing, and the elderly, who often have poor dietary habits, may have increased needs.)

Magnesium ● Although there's little evidence of harm from moderately large doses of this mineral, caution is urged, since scientists are just beginning to study its effects in large doses. *USRDA:* 400 milligrams. *Maximum:* 400 milligrams.

Zinc ● The noticeable side effects of too much zinc can include nausea, vomiting and diarrhea. Yet it's the unseen that may be of more concern. High doses of zinc can create a copper deficiency, a condition that has been shown to increase levels of LDL (low-density lipoprotein) cholesterol (the kind that causes coronary heart disease) in laboratory animals. To be safe, the ratio of zinc to copper should be about 10:1. If your multiple contains, for instance, 20 milligrams of zinc, it should also have 2 milligrams of copper. *USRDA:* 15 milligrams. *Maximum:* 30 milligrams.

No Cold Turkey

If you suspect that you're taking too much of a vitamin or mineral, don't stop completely. "Cut back to about half of your current dosage," says Dr. Vivian. "Your body has adjusted itself to handle a massive dose, so if you stop altogether, it could trigger a deficiency."

As a general rule, Dr. Saltman concludes, it's best to stay below five times the USRDA for minerals and vitamins.

If you're thinking about increasing the dosage of some nutrients, or you're just curious about your present vitamin regimen, it might be wise to consult your doctor or a registered dietitian. This is especially important if you have an illness such as diabetes or high blood pressure, since large doses of some supplements can interfere with the functions of medications.

"It's a multifaceted issue. It's not as simple as popping the top off a bottle and swallowing a few pills," says Dr. Saltman. "The most positive step that people can take is to realize that there is a real potential for harm when taking megadoses of some vitamins and minerals. Once they accept that, they'll be able to objectively look at their personal program and make sure they're on safe ground."

Protecting and Restoring Your Good Health

Sinus Relief Update

Right now 30 to 50 million sinus sufferers probably wish they were fish. Denizens of the deep don't have sinuses, nor is pollen a part of their world. So, unlike humans, they have little trouble with allergy-induced sinus congestion and headaches.

Sinuses are cavities, or hollow air spaces, found all over the body. The ones that concern most people are the paranasal sinuses in the skull. There are four sets: the frontal sinuses, just above the nose behind the eyebrows; the maxillary sinuses, behind each cheekbone; the sphenoid sinuses, behind the nose; and the ethmoid sinuses, behind each side of the bridge of the nose. Each is lined with a mucous membrane and connects to the nasal cavity by narrow passageways.

This is where the plot thickens. When these connecting ducts clog and the sinuses can't drain and exchange air with the nose, they can become inflamed. Air and mucus trapped in an obstructed sinus can become quite painful. When fluids accumulate, bacteria can breed and cause a sinus infection, better known as sinusitis. A headache usually, but not always, results.

It takes very little to gum up the sinus works, as many hay fever sufferers are reminded between mid-August and mid-October (or the first frost), because these are the dreaded ragweed months. Other flora, such as goldenrod, poplar, cottonwood, pigweed, sage and a host of grasses, also send

76

pollen skyward at this time of year, making life miserable for people with allergic noses.

"When an allergen gets inside the nose, certain cells, called 'mast cells,' which are sensitive to the invading agent, react in an almost explosive manner," says Larry Duberstein, M.D., a Memphis rhinologist (nose specialist) and president of the American Rhinologic Society. "This defense mechanism causes inflammation and swelling of the membranes, and the passages close off to keep out more of the allergen. Unfortunately, in this case, too much of what's intended to be a good thing gives negative results and the blockage causes problems."

Pollen is a seasonal allergen but by far not the only instigator of sinus problems. Some people are sensitive to house dust, feathers, wool, animal dander and cotton, to name a few, and are subjected to sinus attacks throughout the year.

Sinus problems can also be caused by a cold or other respiratory illness, which makes mucous membranes swell and nasal secretions thicken. "With a cold or viral infection, you may have some fever and sinus pain for a week or less, and then it subsides," says allergy and immunology specialist John Salvaggio, M.D., chairman of the Department of Medicine at Tulane Medical School, New Orleans, and past president of the American Academy of Allergy and Immunology.

"With allergic reactions, the symptoms last longer and recur. If a person has more than two or three 'colds' a year, there's a good chance he's allergic to something."

Other causes of poor drainage and sinusitis can be a deviated septum (misalignment of the bone and cartilage that separate the nasal passages), polyps in the nose or enlarged adenoids. Bacteria or other infectious organisms can get into the sinus cavities while you're swimming.

But to a person caught in the viselike grip of a sinus headache, relief is more important than cause. The adjective *splitting* is most often used to describe the pain behind the eyebrows when the frontal sinuses are affected. In some cases, the pain may be on only one side, depending on the sinus involved, or it can occur between the nose and eye. In rarer cases, pain is felt in the jaw, teeth, ears, neck and top of the head.

Nose-itis or Sinusitis?

Some people with recurring headaches mistakenly self-diagnose sinuses as the culprit. "A lot of headaches, discomfort and stuffiness are caused by a change in the lining of the nose, usually in response to an allergen," says Anthony Yonkers, M.D., chairman of the Department of Ear, Nose and Throat at the University of Nebraska Medical Center, Omaha. "People use the term 'sinus' generally to refer to a variety of headaches and nasal conditions, but actually 'nose-itis' is a better description of what they really have."

The reason for the confusion is simple, says Dr. Duberstein. "The wall between the nose and sinuses is served by the same nerves, so when there's pain it's often difficult to know whether it's nose or sinus."

Tension headaches are also confused with sinus problems. Throbbing from stress, however, will usually subside when you are lying down, and it doesn't include stuffy nostrils.

The only sure way to tell if you have a sinus problem, adds Dr. Duberstein, is with ultrasound, a CAT scan or x-rays. A family history of sinus problems may be a tip-off, since scientists have found it possible to be genetically predisposed to the condition.

Sinus attacks come in two forms: acute, which come on rapidly, last an extremely painful week or two, then subside for a while; and the less painful chronic attacks that can last months, intensifying when the sensitive sinus membranes encounter the allergen or irritant, such as cigarette smoke, perfume, smog or even some odors that arise from cooking.

"Chronic problems are usually caused by some obstruction of the passages, such as polyps or a deviated septum, or scar tissue from repeated attacks," says Dr. Duberstein.

While most sinus attacks are acute, repeated episodes can cause permanent thickening of the sinus membrane and lead to a chronic problem. Complications are rare but can be serious if left untreated. Ear infections, bronchitis and pneumonia can develop, as can infections of the eye cavity or brain. "Because the sinuses are so close to the brain, infections can lead to very serious, or even life-threatening, complications," Dr. Duberstein adds.

Facing the Enemy

If your sinus problems are caused by allergies, "prevention is a major goal," says Dr. Salvaggio, "and avoiding allergens is the key. If you don't know what you're allergic to, consult a doctor for tests, because it'll save you a lot of pain and discomfort in the long run."

Avoidance once meant packing up and moving, hopefully leaving the allergen behind. Doctors now question that idea. Says Dr. Salvaggio, "We now know that if someone's genetically predisposed to allergic reaction, they'll have problems wherever they go. They may move to an area of the southwest that's free of ragweed and feel great at first, but eventually they may develop an allergic reaction to another pollen."

Misery in a New Month

Similarly, your hay fever symptoms can shift to a different season as your body becomes sensitive to other pollens.

Your doctor may be able to give you a chart that shows the peak pollen seasons for a variety of plants for each region. Many local weather bureaus also offer pollen advisories.

A series of shots is available that desensitizes you to the effects of the allergen. Air conditioners also help, not so much in filtering out allergens but in making the hours inside more comfortable, since the hot days of summer are pollinating times for many varieties of plants, trees and grasses.

If the air is dry, a humidifier keeps nasal passages moist, which helps trap viruses and bacteria that could cause an infection. Air filters, especially the electrostatic type that remove particles from the air better than the traditional fan and filter variety, are a good idea.

Cover heating, cooling and ventilation ducts with dust filters and clean them regularly. Floors should be kept as clean as possible and, ideally, carpet should be avoided because it collects allergens.

"It also helps to know how to blow your nose," says Dr. Yonkers. "You can force infected mucus back into your sinuses by blowing wrong. The right way is to blow gently, without holding your nostril shut."

If you find yourself wracked by the pain of sinus headache,

avoid over-the-counter nose decongestant sprays and drops, says Dr. Duberstein. "The decongestants can paralyze the cilia, or nose hairs, which causes fluids and secretions to collect and just make a bad situation worse."

Beware the Rebound Effect

Another reason to avoid decongestant nose sprays is "rebound congestion." Dr. Duberstein adds, "The sprays give temporary relief, so many people use them constantly. But they find that as the effects wear off, their passages clog up worse than before."

The U.S. Food and Drug Administration recently approved three new prescription sprays that don't cause swelling of sinus passages. Two of the sprays, which contain a form of unabsorbed cortisone, prevent the "explosive" reaction and inflammation that occurs in the nose when an allergen invades. Their generic names are beclomethasone and flunisolide. The other recently approved spray, cromolyn sodium, works by preventing the mast cells from releasing irritating substances into the nose.

"The best nasal spray contains no decongestant," says Dr. Duberstein. "It's a saline solution made at home with ¼ teaspoon of salt and eight ounces of clean water." (Chills or fever and a thick, yellow nasal secretion accompanying sinus pain may point to a bacterial infection, in which case you should see your doctor.)

For some allergic folks, it's easier to get relief by swallowing a pill, which is the reason antihistamines are so popular. These medications reduce swelling and congestion by blocking the release of troublesome histamine, which causes inflammations when released in the nasal passages in response to an allergen.

"In some cases, a physician should be seen first, because the type of antihistamine needed will depend on a variety of factors, such as the patient's body size and allergic condition," says Dr. Duberstein. "When to take the medication is important, too, because it's possible to develop a tolerance with extended use."

Ordinary steam helps because the warmth and moisture loosen stubborn mucus. Ideally, a steam bath is the best source, but many sinus sufferers settle for vaporizers and hot showers. Another option is a warm compress draped across the eyes and cheekbones. A thick washcloth or towel soaked in warm (not hot) water may suffice. Some people achieve best results while sitting and tipping the head slightly forward to help the sinuses drain through the nose, avoiding the nagging postnasal drip in the back of the throat as the mucus begins moving.

Chronic sufferers are finding relief through a new technique called functional endoscopic sinus surgery. A specialist uses a rodlike telescope and tools to clean out blocked drainage passages. The procedure is done in the doctor's office, with a recovery period of about one day, says Dr. Duberstein.

Acetaminophen may also help reduce sinus pain. And in the it-couldn't-hurt category of relief, there are a few suggestions that some doctors discount but that may be worth noting.

● Hot herbal teas, especially fenugreek, anise or horehound.
● Hot chicken soup, which a team of scientists from Mount Sinai Medical Center in Miami Beach actually studied, concluding that the liquid helps induce mucus movement.
● Vitamin C, which some studies have shown has antihistamine qualities.

If all else fails to move the mucus that has your sinuses clogged tighter than a 5 o'clock freeway, you might be able to literally shake it loose. Some determined sinus sufferers have reported beneficial results after jogging, walking and bicycling.

Ulcer Cure: A Revolutionary Approach That Looks Promising

For the millions of Americans who suffer from duodenal ulcer, the most common form of ulcer, doctors can offer little more than a good news/bad news prognosis. The good news: Conventional therapy—drugs that either reduce or neutralize acid or coat the stomach lining—can heal most ulcers in four to six weeks. The bad news: Healing is not curing.

In an estimated 75 to 90 percent of cases, the ulcer recurs. In fact, roughly 10 to 20 percent of those who have surgery for duodenal ulcer still have some symptoms, and in 10 percent the ulcer returns. "There's an old dictum in gastroenterology," says one researcher. " 'Once an ulcer, always an ulcer.' "

But new findings may change all that. Two Australian doctors have isolated bacteria that they think may be responsible for many if not all duodenal ulcers and chronic gastritis. Their theory is that relapse rates are high in ulcer cases because standard treatment never eradicates the ulcer's cause.

Most important, they believe they may also have found a cure that is simple, inexpensive and quick. It involves antibiotics and an over-the-counter medication that most Americans have probably used at some time for upset stomach or traveler's diarrhea.

In 1979, Robin Warren, a pathologist, and Barry Marshall, M.D., a gastroenterologist at the Royal Perth Hospital, discovered that an odd strain of bacteria was present in nearly all the test samples from a group of patients with active chronic gastritis. Gastritis is a condition that frequently precedes or accompanies full-blown duodenal ulcer.

Over the next few years, Dr. Warren and Dr. Marshall tested hundreds of patients with gastritis and duodenal ulcer and in most found this spiral bacteria, which appeared to them to be a form of *campylobacter*. The most common *campylobacter* bacteria is known to cause diarrhea in humans. They named the new strain *Campylobacter pyloridis* because of its location in the stomach near the pylorus, the valve that holds food in the stomach.

At the same time, they began experimenting with a compound that had been shown to heal duodenal ulcer and, in fact, has a lower relapse rate than more conventional treatments. The substance is a compound of a heavy metal called bismuth, which had been used to treat syphilis and other bacterial infections before the discovery of penicillin in the 1940s. A very similar compound is the main ingredient of a common American over-the-counter remedy, Pepto-Bismol.

What Dr. Marshall and Dr. Warren found was that in a surprising number of cases, the bismuth compound worked. For many of the patients, not only did the bacteria disappear but so did their ulcers. In their most recent study, the researchers found that about 30 percent of ulcer patients who took the bismuth compound alone were clear of the bacteria, compared to none in the group given the usual ulcer treatment, cimetidine (Tagamet).

But the best clearance—75 percent—came in the group given the bismuth compound and an antibacterial drug similar to a prescription medication sold in the United States under the trade name Flagyl.

Of course, the real test for any ulcer treatment is the relapse rate. Reports Dr. Marshall, "When we did the relapse study, we found the relapse rate was proportional to the number of patients who still had the germ after treatment. The relapse rate was between 80 and 100 percent in all the Tagamet patients. It was between 50 and 70 percent in the patients who got the bismuth and placebo. But the relapse rate was only about 30 percent in the patients who got the bismuth and antibiotic."

The Tagamet patients were subsequently given the antibiotic and bismuth and, says Dr. Marshall, "they're all well. In fact, we have hardly had any patients requiring further treatment."

How It Works

How does *campylobacter* cause gastritis and duodenal ulcer in the first place? Dr. Marshall and his colleagues believe the bacteria, which can live in the acid environment of the stomach, either digest or in some way damage the mucous lining of the stomach. Without that protective lining, which he describes as "like plastic wrap," acid irritates and eventually eats a hole in the stomach, causing an ulcer.

The bacteria theory may explain why so many ulcers run in families. Scientists have long believed there was some genetic component to ulcers, though the exact connection has never been established. "We don't know how this bacterium is spread," says Dr. Marshall, "but there's some suggestion that it's through kissing, because husbands with duodenal ulcers often have wives who have gastritis. In fact, about half the wives of duodenal ulcer patients have gastritis."

Nevertheless, *Campylobacter pyloridis* does not appear to be highly infectious, though it's been estimated that as many as 40 percent of middle-aged Americans have it (compared to only 10 percent of young adults). Many of them, however, are symptomless.

One of the fortunate aspects of the Australian discovery—technically a rediscovery, since the bacterium was observed and promptly forgotten at least 40 years ago—is that the cure was not far behind. And it is an inexpensive cure. Conventional therapy, which includes indefinite maintenance, can cost roughly $1,000 or more over a period of five years, estimates Dr. Marshall. "And even then you still get a high relapse rate," he says.

Campylobacter pyloridis is very susceptible to the bismuth compound. Even if the antibiotic stops working, as it sometimes does, the bismuth continues to fight the bacteria, says Dr. Marshall. The germs don't seem to build up any immunity to it. And bismuth is easily and inexpensively available in Pepto-Bismol. "A two-week therapy of the bismuth compound and the antibiotic, which is really all that's usually needed, costs around $30," says the researcher. "And with this new therapy we're *curing* around 75 percent of the patients and the treatment doesn't have to go on for months. That's because it's not just a treatment, it's a cure."

Another advantage is the lack of significant side effects, though Dr. Marshall cautions that none of the *campylobacter* studies, including his own, have been large or long enough to rule out possible side effects. He has now undertaken a clinical trial using the bismuth/antibiotic treatment on nonulcer dyspepsia, a related digestive disorder in which victims have gastritis without ulcer. "We want to see if we can prevent a relapse of nonulcer dyspepsia in exactly the same way as we prevent relapse of duodenal ulcer," he says.

Though other researchers have had some success with Pepto-Bismol alone, Dr. Marshall found that the bacteria tended to recolonize in many cases, so the one-two punch of bismuth and antibiotic appears to be necessary to eradicate the bug totally.

No Treatment Yet

Needless to say, the Australian findings have been causing a stir in the gastroenterological community since the first study appeared in the prestigious British journal *Lancet.*

But the Australian studies, while intriguing to the medical community, are still preliminary. Though the work is promising, Pepto-Bismol and antibiotics are unlikely to become the treatment of choice overnight. They represent a revolutionary treatment for ulcer, which up until this point has been attacked from one direction: acid reduction.

"This is a fresh breeze, a new direction," says Frank Lanza, M.D., of Baylor College of Medicine in Houston, who did a study in which a two- to three-week dose of Pepto-Bismol alone healed and prevented the recurrence of gastritis in a small group of patients. "We are finally getting away from the 'acid is everything' thinking. We couldn't keep attacking this problem in the same old ways. We could heal ulcers, but the only way to prevent recurrence was to keep giving patients drugs indefinitely. Although ulcer drugs like cimetidine are relatively innocuous, they do have some systemic side effects."

The Australians have done more than simply stand by their work. In fact, Dr. Marshall was so convinced of the connection between this new bacterium and gastritis and ulcer, he swallowed a colony of *Campylobacter pyloridis* himself as a test, developed gastritis and cured it with a dose of bismuth and antibiotic.

These days, some of the big guns in gastroenterology are starting to pay attention, which could spell relief earlier than expected for ulcer and gastritis sufferers. "There are some very serious people involved in this research now," says Dr. Lanza.

More Ulcer Help from the Drugstore

While the Pepto-Bismol ulcer cure is still under investigation, there may be another alternative that's also as close as the pharmacy shelf.

Researchers have found that the regular daily use of the common antacid Maalox can prevent the relapse of duodenal ulcers.

In a multicenter study, researchers used a form of Maalox

called Maalox TC, which has 2½ to 3 times the acid-buffering capacity of regular Maalox, on a group of duodenal ulcer patients.

Out of 173 patients with healed ulcers, only 25 percent had a recurrence within a year after taking three tablets every morning and night, according to one of the researchers, Chesley Hines, M.D., of the Ochsner Clinic in New Orleans. The greatest benefit was reaped by smokers in the study. "It's been shown clearly that ulcers recur more frequently in smokers, so it would make sense that a program to prevent recurrence would benefit smokers the most," explains Dr. Hines.

The researchers compared the Maalox TC to both cimetidine and a placebo (dummy pill) and, while the cimetidine users had only a slightly higher recurrence rate, there is less risk of side effects with the Maalox TC.

Maalox TC is readily available over the counter. Unlike the Pepto-Bismol/antibiotic treatment, though, it must be taken regularly.

Warning: This Star Causes Cancer

When was the last time you sunbathed? Was it last Labor Day weekend at the beach? That warm Indian summer day at the lake? Or during your midwinter cruise to the Caribbean? Are you sure that's all?

Have you taken into account the morning you shoveled an overnight snowfall out of your driveway? Or the hour you spent shopping at the outdoor flea market? Or the 45 minutes you watched the kids at the playground?

You didn't think of those times, did you? Most people don't. And those may be just the times—when you don't realize you're spending too much time in the sun—that you're exposing your vulnerable skin to an extra dose of ultraviolet light that could lead to skin cancer.

"I have a patient, a schoolteacher, who told me she didn't spend much time in the sun," says Henry E. Wiley III, M.D., assistant professor of medicine at the University of South Florida, Tampa, and a dermatologist in private practice. "I could tell that wasn't the case by the tan on her forearms. It turned out she spends 45 minutes every school day supervising the children at recess. She thought that because she wasn't out playing tennis and golf at midday that she wasn't getting any sun. We may be exposed to hundreds of hours of incidental sun that we don't count."

In the United States, dermatologists and other skin cancer experts have their work cut out for them. Despite the fact that skin cancer is epidemic—with roughly half a million new cases a year—most Americans still consider tanned skin a sign of health. In fact, when researchers at the University of Florida in Gainesville surveyed a group of 100 mothers, they found that most associated premature wrinkling and skin cancer with overexposure to sunlight, yet 75 percent of them felt a tan looked healthy and attractive. Only half used sunscreens on themselves and their children on any regular basis.

Stay Out of the Sun

Ironically, with the use of sunscreens and a few other precautions, skin cancer is almost entirely preventable. All you really have to do is avoid the sun.

Most basal cell and squamous cell carcinomas—the most common and curable skin cancers—are caused by overexposure to the ultraviolet radiation of the sun, primarily the rays designated UVB. These short-wavelength rays are most prevalent between 10:00 A.M. and 2:00 P.M. (11:00 A.M. and 3:00 P.M. daylight saving time) in most parts of the country.

While UVB rays are tanning, burning and wrinkling your skin, they can scramble your skin cells' DNA—vital genetic material—causing cancer to develop.

The most virulent form of skin cancer is malignant melanoma, which is responsible for 75 percent of all skin cancer deaths and roughly 2 to 3 percent of all cancer deaths nationwide. The incidence of melanoma is growing at a faster rate than that of any other kind of cancer, except lung cancer in women.

Until recently, scientists weren't sure the sun's radiation

had much to do with malignant melanoma. Now there is some convincing circumstantial evidence that sun exposure—particularly the shorter, more intense exposures of the recreational sunbather rather than the long-term occupational exposures of, for instance, farmers and fishermen—may be linked to the disease.

Melanoma patients tend to be much younger, by 10 to 20 years, than patients with the more common basal cell carcinoma, which tends to develop after age 35 from the effects of a lifetime of sun exposure. Arthur Sober, M.D., of the Harvard Medical School, and Robert Lew, Ph.D., of the University of Massachusetts Medical Center, in a study released last spring, also found that people who had had blistering sunburns as adolescents were twice as likely to develop melanoma—with poor tanners at highest risk.

Clearly, the time to prevent this deadly form of cancer is early. But a study headed by Robert S. Stern, M.D., of Beth Israel Hospital and Harvard Medical School in Boston, found that it's really never too late. Dr. Stern and his colleagues, examining the data from a number of long-term skin cancer studies, estimate that the simple use of sunscreens with high sun protection factor (SPF) numbers in childhood could reduce the risk of basal cell and squamous cell carcinomas by 78 percent and might lower the risk of malignant melanoma over a lifetime. But all is not lost if you were a sun-worshipper as a child, as long as you avoid the sun as an adult, says Dr. Stern. Your risk of developing a nonmelanoma skin cancer may be reduced by 88 to 91 percent if you avoid the sun or use a sunscreen now.

Sun Smarts

To help you get started on your skin cancer prevention course, we asked the experts for some specific advice. Here's what they suggest.

Keep a Sun Log ● Dr. Wiley counsels his patients to write down all the times they're exposed to the sun, on purpose or inadvertently. The beach isn't the only place you're likely to get a sunburn. You can get a first-class burn on a ski trip. At those high elevations there's less atmosphere to filter the sun's rays and, like the sand and water at the beach, snow reflects ultraviolet light. (In fact snow, white-painted surfaces and aluminum reflect more ultraviolet light than sand: 70 to 90 percent compared to about 25 percent.)

Wear a Sunscreen Daily, No Matter What You're Doing ● That advice is being given to thousands of participants in two long-term studies supported by the National Cancer Institute now being done at the University of Arizona at Tucson. (Tucson is the skin cancer capital of the United States, and second only to Queensland, Australia, in the incidence of melanoma.) "We tell the patients to put their sunscreen on first thing in the morning," says Lynn Ferro, clinic coordinator. "It should become a habit, like brushing your teeth. That way you never forget." Most experts advise using a sunscreen with an SPF of 15—it's marked on the package—and to put it on anywhere from 15 minutes to two hours before sun exposure for maximum benefit. Also, pay close attention to the application directions. Studies show most people put on too thin a layer.

Wear Proper Clothing ● Most experts advise keeping covered up as much as possible when you're likely to do a little too much baking in the sun. But what kind of clothing should you wear?

"Unfortunately, it's not possible to go into a store and pick out a shirt or hat with an SPF rating," says Dr. Wiley. "My best advice is to take the hat or article of clothing and hold it up to the light. The more you can see through it, the less protection you're going to have." As a rule of thumb, cotton clothing tends to be more protective than synthetic fabrics, and dark shades more effective than light ones.

Eat More Yellow and Green Vegetables and Fruits ● There's no conclusive evidence yet, but the vitamin A and beta-carotene in these vegetables and fruits may help prevent skin cancer. That's one of the things they're investigating in the Tucson study. Thomas Moon, Ph.D., the principal investigator, says vitamin A was chosen because of some suggestive evidence that it can prevent cancer, specifically epithelial cancers such as skin cancer. Though the Tucson studies are far from over, Dr. Moon says, some participants, who were chosen because they have precancerous skin changes called actinic keratoses, have reported some improvement.

Beware the Skin Cancer Myths ● You don't have to be blond-haired and blue-eyed to get skin cancer, though your risks are greater if you are. About a quarter of the patients in Dr. Moon's study have midtone, olive or dark complexions. There is evidence that those people develop skin cancers in the same way as their fairer counterparts, "but it takes a larger dose of sun," says Dr. Moon.

And, although most nonmelanoma skin cancers can be cured (even melanomas have a high cure rate when caught early), skin cancer is not a disease to be taken lightly. Having a skin cancer removed is not like having the tartar scraped off your teeth. Skin cancer is a serious disease and there tends to be a high rate of recurrence.

Filter Trouble Out of Your Bloodstream

Blood clots can really throw a monkey wrench into your machinery. A clot that lodges in the arteries feeding your heart muscles causes a heart attack. A clot that travels to your neck or head can induce a stroke. One that settles in your lungs creates a pulmonary embolism, a kind of "heart attack of the lungs" that's as deadly as the real thing.

Small clots, called microemboli, can form in capillaries and cause kidney, eye and nerve damage. People with diabetes, who are particularly at risk for diseases of the small and large blood vessels, sometimes face having toes or even a leg amputated because their circulation has gotten so poor the limb has died.

So, counting the 20 digits on your hands and feet, there

are plenty of good reasons to keep your blood flowing smoothly. But how can you do that?

Lifesaver Gone Awry

Clots develop when flat, disk-shaped cell fragments in the blood, called platelets, are "activated." This means they are triggered to stick together (platelet aggregation) and to stick to blood vessel walls (platelet adhesion). We are grateful this occurs when we're spilling blood after an accident, for clotting can stop bleeding in seconds. But this same process, if it goes awry, can be life-threatening.

Topping most hematologists' list of clot causers is blood vessel damage. This can be from fatty deposits caused by high blood fat levels. Or it can be microscopic damage, usually caused by the rapid, turbulent flow of blood near a bend or fork in the artery. High blood pressure is the main cause here.

This damage attracts platelets like flies to honey. When they come in contact with the injured area, platelets change their characteristics drastically. They begin to swell and to take on an irregular shape, with numerous protruding "feet," or pseudopods. They become sticky so that they cling to the collagen fibers in the damaged vessel. And they secrete large quantities of biochemicals that activate more platelets, causing an ever-growing pileup that attracts white blood cells and more fat. Before you know it, a once free-flowing artery has become a bottleneck.

Fortunately, there are things you can do to keep such a scenario from happening. Strictly speaking, you can't actually thin your blood, but you can alter its readiness to clot.

"The first things I tell people are, 'Don't smoke, lower your fat intake, keep your weight and blood pressure down, avoid salt, exercise regularly and, if you have diabetes, keep your blood sugar normal,' " says Arthur Vinik, M.D., professor of internal medicine and surgery at the University of Michigan at Ann Arbor and a specialist in diabetes. "All these things help normalize platelet function and prevent blood vessel disease."

Then, as a second line of defense, you may want to consider other factors that affect platelet action.

Aspirin's Intriguing Role

Researchers started looking at aspirin's effect on blood clotting when they saw that people who took a lot of aspirin, such as those with rheumatoid arthritis, had fewer heart attacks than average.

In the 1970s, scientists began studying whether anticlotting properties of aspirin could stop second heart attacks or strokes in high-risk people. In 1985, after reviewing seven studies, federal health officials announced that taking one aspirin (about 325 milligrams) a day could help some heart attack victims reduce the likelihood of a second attack.

Aspirin is known to do two things. It blocks an enzyme in platelets that produces a biochemical called thromboxane, which makes platelets clump together and causes blood vessel constriction. The problem is that the same enzyme is also present in blood vessel walls and is used to produce a biochemical called prostacyclin, which has exactly the opposite effect—it unclumps platelets and dilates blood vessels.

But platelets appear to be more sensitive to aspirin than the blood vessel walls are. So researchers believe that fairly small amounts of aspirin will work to inhibit thromboxane formation while leaving prostacyclin production unaffected. In a study by researchers at the University of Minnesota, as little as 20 milligrams a day (one-quarter of a children's aspirin tablet) inhibited thromboxane formation. Most previous studies had used up to 1,000 milligrams a day.

There's little agreement among experts as to the "ideal" amount of aspirin to take to stop clotting. And researchers point out that studies have yet to show that aspirin can prevent a first heart attack or stroke, although there is research in progress that may one day prove that. In addition, studies that looked at aspirin's benefits in circulation-related diabetic disorders have so far proved disappointing.

"Research is now showing that aspirin may do some good and some harm," says hematology researcher Daniel Deykin, M.D., a Boston University professor of medicine and biochemistry. Some intestinal bleeding almost always occurs with aspirin. And if you're taking aspirin and have a heart attack, doctors may not give you anticoagulants, fearing you may have excessive bleeding. And although aspirin studies *do* show a trend toward fewer heart attacks, they do not show reduced death rates. In other words, aspirin may *not* prevent fatal heart attacks.

"We need to avoid premature enthusiasm for any one mode of therapy until clinical trials establish clear benefits," Dr. Deykin says.

Omega-3 May Stop Clots

Researchers thought there was something unusual going on when they discovered that, despite their high fat intake, Eskimos had little heart disease. The answer seemed to lie in their diet, which was mostly fish.

Investigation showed that certain cold-water fish contain omega-3 fatty acids. Studies have shown that a diet rich in these fats reduces the number of blood platelets and reduces platelet aggregation. Omega-3's interfere with platelets' manufacture of thromboxane, leading to the production of a much less potent form of thromboxane.

That effect in itself would probably be enough to limit clotting. But omega-3's have another effect. They also accumulate in the cells lining the artery walls. These cells make anticlotting prostacyclin, and omega-3 fatty acids are readily converted into prostacyclin.

Both these actions may help prevent heart disease in its early stages, researchers speculate. The benefits of omega-3's are probably best seen when you substitute fish for foods high in saturated fat, like beef and dairy products, Dr. Vinik says. That's advice he gives his patients with diabetes.

Mackerel, salmon, trout, tuna and sardines are richest in omega-3's.

Exercise Can Help

Doctors know that patients confined to bed after surgery are more likely to form blood clots in their legs, clots that can break loose, travel to their lungs and cause serious damage. Even a few hours of immobilization, such as a long drive in a car, can increase clotting activity.

One reason this happens is that blood often clots when it

flows very slowly through blood vessels, for small amounts of coagulants are always being formed. These are generally removed from the blood by cells in the liver. If the blood is flowing too slowly, concentrations of coagulants in local areas often rise high enough to initiate clotting. But when the blood flows rapidly, they are quickly mixed with large quantities of blood and are removed during passage though the liver.

So it might seem possible that the opposite of inactivity — exercise — would make blood less likely to clot. That's exactly what Finnish researchers found to be the case.

They looked at platelet aggregation in middle-aged, overweight men with mildly elevated blood pressure. The men were put on a 12-week exercise program of brisk walking and slow jogging five times a week, for 45 to 60 minutes per session. At the end of the program, the men had a 27 to 36 percent reduction in platelet aggregation compared to a similar control group of men whose physical activity level remained stable. In the exercising men, platelets had become less sensitive to the biochemicals that make them clot. This reduced sensitivity lasted for several days after exercise *(Circulation)*.

Dr. Vinik points out that strenuous, nonaerobic exercise, such as weight lifting, can have the opposite effect. "A short, intense burst of nonaerobic exercise is a great way to *activate* platelets. Gentle, regular aerobic exercise is much better." Such exercise can also help permanently normalize blood sugar levels. That's something Dr. Vinik feels is crucial for maintaining healthy blood vessels.

A Folk Remedy Vindicated

Garlic has been used for centuries as a tonic for heart ailments. Russians downed an infusion of garlic and vodka to fight poor circulation. The French fed it to horses suffering from blood clots in the legs. And modern-day chemical analysis is proving folk medicine to be right on target.

"Clinical studies seem to be pretty much in agreement that there's something in garlic that helps prevent blood clotting," says Eric Block, Ph.D., chairman and professor of the Department of Chemistry at the State University of New York at Albany. Dr. Block has been looking at the components in garlic that work specifically as anticlotting agents.

The most active ingredient they've found so far is a compound they call ajoene (from the Spanish *ajo,* which means "garlic"). "Ajoene seems to change the surface membrane of platelet cells so that they're less likely to stick together. It may also affect the platelets' ability to produce thromboxane, a chemical that causes clumping. Other compounds in garlic may also influence thromboxane production," Dr. Block says. Ajoene is not yet available commercially.

Right now, the best way to take advantage of garlic's blood-thinning effects is to eat whole bulbs, Dr. Block says. Prepared garlic preparations are less likely to have anticlotting action.

"Certainly, evidence suggests that garlic is very healthy," Dr. Block says. "The only side effect it seems to have is bad breath. If you're a hermit, I'd advise you to eat lots and lots of garlic."

You might also want to load up on onions, which seem to have similar, although less potent, chemical properties, Dr. Block says.

If you have to face people, get them to indulge, too. Eating garlic and onions saturates the cells in the nose with these molecules, so they can't smell your breath—or their own, for that matter.

Benefits from Vitamin E?

Like aspirin and fish oil, vitamin E may affect platelet function a number of ways. Studies are mixed, though. Some show positive results; some don't. Vitamin E may take a long time to work, its effects may be relatively weak, and it may have no effect at all in people whose platelet function is normal.

During platelet aggregation, a chemical reaction called lipid peroxidation takes place. This process creates unstable molecular particles called free radicals that may promote more aggregation.

Because vitamin E helps to neutralize free radical particles and lowers levels of lipid peroxides, it may suppress platelet activity in some people, especially those with abnormally high levels of blood fats.

Vitamin E may work best in protecting the blood vessel

wall's ability to manufacture prostacyclin, the biochemical that helps to prevent platelets from sticking to blood vessels. In a study from Krakow, Poland, rabbits fed a diet high in saturated fat had a 90 percent decrease in arterial generation of prostacyclin. But when vitamin E was added to the same high-fat diet, the prostacyclin-generating system in arteries was fully protected.

Studies done by Manfred Steiner, M.D., Ph.D., professor of medicine, Division of Hematology at Brown University, Providence, Rhode Island, show similar effects in humans.

Dr. Steiner had a group of people take 400 international units or more of vitamin E a day for several weeks. Then he examined how likely their platelets were to stick to collagen, a tissue found on damaged artery surfaces. He found they were much less sticky.

Looking at both normal and vitamin E-enriched platelets under an electron microscope, he saw a distinct difference. "When they come in contact with collagen, platelets not enriched with vitamin E send out long spiny projections [pseudopods] to anchor themselves to the collagen," Dr. Steiner says. In contrast, vitamin E-rich platelets send out very few pseudopods. "The pictures we saw were amazing, very striking," Dr. Steiner says. "The sharp reduction in pseudopods makes good sense to explain the platelets' decreased adhesiveness."

He believes vitamin E may be the perfect partner for aspirin in people with clotting problems. "The two together may be a very good combination, because vitamin E inhibits the very first step, which is adhesion, and aspirin would then inhibit the following step, aggregation. I think there is good potential for clinical application, and that this combination should be further studied."

A Rejuvenation
Approach to Arthritis

From the Arthritis Foundation

If you're among the one million people who develop arthritis each year, you know that getting up and exercising while your joints ache can be trying. But think about your car after it sits idle for a few weeks. The engine may not want to crank right up and probably needs a little coaxing, but it runs great after it warms up.

In the words of Frederic C. McDuffie, M.D., who is vice-president of medical affairs for the Arthritis Foundation, "People with arthritis *must* exercise their joints daily to ensure adequate joint mobility and muscle strength. An exercise program that's properly designed and implemented can keep joints flexible, help maintain muscle strength, build overall stamina, lead to a more positive self-image and create a sense of accomplishment."

Nowhere is the adage "use it or lose it" more apropos than with arthritis. "The longer you sit around in pain doing nothing, the worse it gets," says Michele Boutaugh, Arthritis Foundation vice-president for patient services. "You get stiffer and stiffer, and eventually you can lose the use of the affected joint."

If you need more convincing, just ask any of the 60 people who took part in a research project at the University of Missouri. They ranged in age from 21 to 83 and all had rheumatoid arthritis and osteoarthritis in their legs and feet. As part of the project, they did some water jogging—moving their legs in a jogging motion while in deep water. Since their bodies were lighter in the water, there was less strain on their leg and foot joints, and they were able to exercise and strengthen weak muscles. They also walked on dry land three days a week for about 30 minutes each day, says project researcher Marion Minor of the University of Missouri-Columbia School of Medicine.

After 12 weeks, their endurance and aerobic power improved, and some had less stiffness and weakness with more joint mobility. In other words, they were on the way to preventing or delaying the crippling deformities sometimes caused by arthritis, and they were leading fuller, more active lives, says Minor.

The Definition of Exercise

Some people believe that "exercise" includes normal daily activities, such as housework, climbing stairs, bending and lifting, or walking. These activities may maintain and improve endurance and muscle tone, and they are fine. But there are some special exercises quite unlike any others, exercises that work specifically on joints. These are the range-of-motion exercises that are the backbone of your exercise program. Range-of-motion exercises help keep joints loose, improve muscle strength and help restore movement that's been lost.

One of the more common range-of-motion exercises for aching hips calls for you to lie on your back with your legs straight and about six inches apart. Point your toes up. Slide one leg out to the side and then back. Try to keep your toes pointing up, and then repeat the exercise with your other leg.

A good range-of-motion exercise for arthritis in the shoulders is to stay on your back and raise one arm over your head, keeping your elbow straight. Keep your arm close to your ear. Return your arm slowly to your side and repeat the movement with your other arm.

(Your physician or therapist will be able to give you more exercises specifically suited to the parts of your body affected by arthritis.)

When doing any of these range-of-motion exercises, move the joint until you feel some pain, hold it there a moment, then move it a wee bit further. If there's slight pain in the joint, be gentle as you move it through whatever motion is possible. Sometimes you may need help, but try to perform as many as possible yourself. If you have a helper, he or she shouldn't use force when helping you with the movements. If possible, do five to ten repetitions per exercise.

A complete exercise program will also include strengthening exercises, because weak muscles add to joint problems. These

GETTING STARTED

If you're one of the 37 million people who suffer from arthritis and you're anxious to begin an exercise program, don't run out and start doing jumping jacks. "Before you start exercising, check with your physician," says Frederic C. McDuffie, M.D., vice-president of medical affairs for the Arthritis Foundation. "Too much exercise can be as harmful as too little. Your doctor, working with a physical or occupational therapist, can help you design a program specifically for your needs."

Another note of caution: If you're in the chronic phase of arthritis, where there's been joint destruction and intense flare-ups despite medication and other treatments, exercise only under the close supervision of your physician and your therapist. The wrong kind of physical activity may put too much strain on weakened joints and lead to permanent damage.

If your doctor gives his blessing, you might want to adopt a new attitude before beginning. Don't think of yourself as a patient trying to overcome a disease. Just as a ballet dancer performs special exercises to strengthen legs and feet, or a pianist practices to keep fingers and arms in shape, you are using exercise to get your joints in better condition.

"You are about to face what may be the biggest challenge of your life—asserting your will upon your body to modify and correct the effects of what could become a serious, disabling condition. A positive frame of mind is a good place to start," says Dr. McDuffie.

Once you've created your exercise program, write it down and keep an exercise diary. In a few months, you can look back on it and see how far you've progressed.

exercises can help maintain or increase muscle strength while putting as little stress on joints as possible.

Isometric exercises have the advantage of causing little joint stress. Basically you're using your muscles to pull or push against a stationary object, which can be anything from a wall to a body part to an exercise belt. Place your hands on a wall and push. You can feel your arm muscles working but there's no joint movement. Another example is to sit in a chair and

START WITH A STRETCH

You must get your body—specifically your aching joints—slowly prepared for exercise, so make stretching the first step before each workout. Here's one example of a safe, slow stretch: While lying in bed, stretch one arm up and then the other. Push your arms forward while opening your hands wide, then pull your arms back and close your hands. For your legs, pull your knees up toward your midsection, do a few slow bicycle turns, then stretch your legs out straight.

Besides preparing you for your daily exercises, such activity also helps prevent morning stiffness. It's similar to what a cat does when it gets up. Also, to avoid injury and reduce stiffness or soreness the next day, it's a good idea to stretch as part of your cooling-down process each time you finish exercising.

To ease any pre-exercise discomfort, you can apply mild heat (it's not necessary that it be really hot) to help relax joints and muscles. It can be a warm bath or whirlpool, a shower or hand-held massage unit so you can aim the water at painful joints, an electric heating pad, a hot water bottle or hot packs. You can even stand next to a heater or radiator. In any case, about 20 minutes should be enough in most cases.

Some people find that cold offers better relief than heat. A plastic bag of ice is the standard method, although a package of frozen vegetables in a towel will do if there's no ice in the freezer. About 10 to 15 minutes is usually enough.

Other people find relief in both hot and cold, and prefer a contrast bath. Soak hands or feet in warm water (about 110°F) for about three minutes, then soak them in cold water (about 65°F) for a minute. Repeat the process three times, and end the treatment with a warm-water soak.

place your right hand on your right knee. Press your knee against your hand while allowing no movement of the arm or leg.

You need not do many isometric exercises to receive the benefits. Each routine held for a count of six seconds, three to four times a day, is enough.

Regenerating Body and Mind

While doing the range-of-motion and strengthening exercises that help get your body—specifically your joints—in shape, you'll probably be standing in the same spot. To prevent boredom and to help build your morale, it often helps to incorporate some type of recreational exercise into your workout. These exercises can include any form of movement, amusement or relaxation that refreshes you physically and mentally and takes your mind off your arthritis. Even active hobbies and crafts are fine.

Your recreational exercises can be done alone or, better yet, in a group, which is a great way to fuel your determination. Consider walking, dancing, swimming, exercising in a pool or doing some other activity that uses both legs and arms, and you'll be enhancing your state of mind *plus* increasing your joint range of motion and improving muscle strength and endurance.

There are five keys to a successful exercise program.

1. Maintain a proper pace. Begin at a comfortable level and gradually increase the number of repetitions to avoid unnecessary pain. Use slow and steady rhythms, relax your muscles for about 10 to 15 seconds between repetitions, and breathe deeply and rhythmically as you exercise. Never hold your breath.

2. Balance your exercise with periods of rest and relaxation. The discomfort caused by arthritis can drain your energy and tire you faster than an exerciser without arthritis would be drained. Consequently, that means you'll need more rest than exercisers who don't have arthritis. Getting enough whole-body rest doesn't mean you have to go to bed and stay there, however. Strive for a balance of rest and activity. During a flare-up you'll need more frequent and longer periods of rest than when your arthritis is quiet. Most physicians recommend 10 to 12 hours of rest for each 24-hour period, divided between actual nighttime sleeping and short periods of lying down and napping during the day.

3. Plan to exercise twice daily for the rest of your life, unless the pain is too severe, in which case contact your physician. In most cases, though, miss a day only if you must and not because you're too busy or in the wrong frame of mind. If you have to skip several days, start again at a slightly lower level.

4. Find a specific time and place and make exercise a daily routine. At first, you might try exercising at different times of the day until you decide what's best for you. Some people find that exercise first thing in the day reduces their morning stiffness.

5. Exercise when you have the least pain and stiffness and when you're not tired. If you're taking a prescription pain medication, plan to do your workout when the drug is having the most effect. Even if there's slight pain, you need to do the range-of-motion exercises to keep your joints loose. If the joint is hot, inflamed, swollen, red or tender to the touch, move it gently through its range of motion. If in doubt, contact your doctor or therapist to find out how to adapt your exercises.

Marathons Are Out

Avoid activities that strain joints, such as weight lifting and running. Jogging is probably out also, but it depends on what your doctor or therapist says. Bicycling depends on the condition of the joints in your legs and hips, and on the terrain. Riding a stationary bike may be better because you can adjust the tension on the wheel to put less strain on your lower extremities.

Avoid chills, too, because they can cause muscles and joints to stiffen. Wear warm clothing and don't exercise in a drafty or cold room. If swimming or exercising in a pool, the water temperature should be 83° to 88°F.

You can calm some fears that may crop up early in your exercise program by learning to listen to your body. During the first few weeks, your body's normal responses to exercise can include increased depth and rate of breathing, increased heart rate, feeling or hearing your heartbeat, mild to moderate sweating and mild muscle aches and tenderness.

If exercise-induced pain lasts longer than two hours, or if the next day your symptoms are worse in the joints you exercised, then you've done too much. Next time cut back or exercise less strenuously. Setbacks aren't permanent. If necessary, find a different exercise that will give you the same results. But make sure the pain is exercise-induced and not caused by some other activity, such as kneeling in the garden or pushing furniture around a room.

Immediately stop exercising if there's tightness or pain in your chest, shortness of breath, dizziness, muscle pain or cramping, or if you're suddenly sick to your stomach. Another signal to stop is extremely sharp pain or more pain than normal—your body is warning you.

When you've finished for the day, you may feel a bit sore. It's not uncommon for you to go at it with a bit too much vigor and need to take either your prescribed pain medication or aspirin. Don't depend only on a pill for pain relief each time, though. If there's so much pain that you need medication after each workout, modify your program.

Above all, don't exclude the other key ingredients necessary to keep arthritis on the run. "Exercise can do wonderful things for people with arthritis, but we must realize that it's only one part of a total arthritis-care program," says Dr. McDuffie. "Your program must also include a physician's continued care, education, medication, rest, joint protection and, for some people, splints. Saving your energy whenever possible, using heat and cold for discomfort and making sure you get proper nutrition are also crucial."

Improvement will—and should be—gradual, but the results will be well worth the work and wait.

LOOKING FOR ANSWERS TO STOP THE PAIN

The Arthritis Foundation is the only voluntary health agency working to find answers for the more than 100 arthritis-related diseases. Research is the foundation's top national priority, with scientists searching for the causes, the cures and ways to prevent the various diseases known as arthritis. The foundation is almost totally privately supported, with funds raised by 71 chapters throughout the nation used to support services and education for people with arthritis, health professionals and the general public.

The Healing Herbs: How to Choose Them and Use Them

When you have a headache, you can either take two aspirins or munch on some willow bark.

It's silly, of course. You wouldn't gnaw on a tree limb to get rid of a headache. But you wouldn't be barking up the wrong tree if you looked to the willow for headache relief.

Concealed within the willow bark is an active pain reliever called salicin. We'll never know who was the first to make the discovery, but for centuries, willow bark has been brewed by people of many cultures as a tea for headaches, rheumatism and fever. The aspirin we buy at the supermarket is a slightly modified, synthetic version of the age-old folk remedy. And aspirin is only one of many over-the-counter (OTC) drugs with herbal roots.

Despite the convenience of commercial OTCs, some people prefer the old herbal cures simply because there's nothing synthetic about them. Why?

"A certain segment of the population has lost faith with the chemical era and they're afraid of the side effects of drugs," says R. F. Chandler, Ph.D., professor of pharmacy at Dalhousie University in Halifax, Nova Scotia, and a member of Canada's Expert Advisory Committee on Herbs and Botanical Preparations.

But just because herbs are natural doesn't mean they're necessarily better or safer than commercial drugs.

"There are two major problems with herbs," says Dr. Chandler. "First, most of us aren't trained to diagnose symptoms of illness. If you start following your own hunches, herbal treatments may or may not have any benefit. But our major fear is that by diagnosing and treating yourself, you may delay detection of serious illness well beyond the point where conventional drugs can help you.

"Second, in spite of the fact that herbs are natural, they aren't all without the possibility of harm. God knows, nicotine is natural, but it's not safe."

Despite the fears, many herbs are safe if used in moderate amounts, in conjunction with a medical diagnosis. But how is the herbal novice to separate the wheat from the chaff, the licorice root from the deadly nightshade? What's safe and effective, and what isn't? And in those cases where an herb is good for you, how much is too much of a good thing?

We asked these questions of several pharmaceutical experts and came up with some practical answers. Here is a list of some of the most effective herbal remedies, along with recommendations for safe "doses."

A Migraine Fighter and a Cough Remedy

These two herbs may help relieve common physical ailments.

Feverfew ● Despite its name, this natural remedy doesn't cool your fevered brow. But it might make what's under your brow feel better, especially if you suffer from migraine headaches.

Patients at the London Migraine Clinic recently put feverfew through its paces. Of the 17 patients, 8 were given capsules of feverfew, while 9 received placebos (dummy pills). None of the patients knew which capsule he or she was taking, the feverfew or the placebo. Doctors selected these patients because they were known to have been taking feverfew on their own.

By the end of the six-month study, the patients receiving feverfew had suffered far fewer migraines than the patients taking a placebo—averaging about 1.50 migraines per month for the feverfew group and 3.43 a month for the placebo group. What's more, after the study, all the patients taking feverfew were weaned off the herb. Their migraine frequency increased dramatically.

Though it still isn't known how feverfew blocks migraine attacks, researchers speculate that substances in the plant appear to make smooth muscle cells less responsive to certain body chemicals that trigger migraine muscle spasms *(British Medical Journal)*.

These findings don't suggest that all migraineurs can toss aside their conventional drugs, though feverfew does seem to help some migraine sufferers. How much feverfew should a person take, and in what form?

"If you take feverfew by eating the leaves, it should be in very small doses—from 50 to 60 milligrams, which is three or four of the little feverfew leaves each day," suggests Varro E. Tyler, Ph.D., dean of the Schools of Pharmacy, Nursing and Health Sciences at Purdue University in Indiana. "Commercial preparations—capsules, for example—are hard to find, but some botanical wholesalers list them."

Some migraineurs who take feverfew mix it into foods to hide the herb's characteristic bitter taste.

Licorice ● If you've taken commercial cough syrups, you might have benefited unknowingly from licorice, which has been used in cough remedies for generations. Licorice is a natural expectorant, which helps you clear out congestion.

But the use of licorice root as a medicinal herb really dates back 4,000 years. Licorice was believed to help relieve stomach pain and mouth ulcers then, and there's some clinical evidence supporting that view today.

"The plant itself has very definite therapeutic effects," says Dr. Chandler. "Basically, it is a reasonably safe plant. But it does cause retention of water, which leads to retention of salt, which in turn leads to high blood pressure."

For this reason, you would be wise to moderate your intake of licorice if you have high blood pressure or heart disease. Too much licorice can lead to potentially dangerous heart rhythms. It is also not a good idea to eat much licorice if you are taking corticosteroid medications, since these drugs also cause water retention. Together, the herb and the drug can be double trouble.

If you don't have high blood pressure and you aren't taking steroid drugs, licorice might be a useful natural remedy for coughs, stomach pain or mouth ulcers. Its use is also being explored in the control of oral herpes, or cold sores, and certain skin cancers, but the clinical evidence supporting its value in these areas is sketchy, at best.

How much licorice to take, then? More to the point, how much not to take?

"About a half a pound of candy a day is bad," says Dr. Chandler, "and most people aren't going to take nearly that much. The real danger is chewing tobacco. Ninety percent of the licorice imported into the United States is used to flavor tobacco."

Nevertheless, Dr. Chandler recommends you restrict your intake of licorice to "small amounts." The traditional amount for congestion is about two grams, adds Dr. Tyler—less than ⅒ ounce, or about a three-inch-long piece of root—as needed.

By the way, if you eat licorice candy, it might not be licorice at all, but anise. If you want the real thing, check the ingredients.

Soothing Herbs for Body and Mind

Here are some herbs that have calmative effects, both physically and mentally.

Capsicum ● You probably know this hot-stuff herb best as chili pepper. Eat too much, and you might think your smoldering stomach would set off the smoke detector. But tummy torch it isn't. Capsicum has been used for years as a "stomachic" or a "carminative"—a medicine that eases stomach pain and flatulence. Capsicum also has been used for diarrhea, cramps and toothache, and you'll find it in some OTC laxatives and in some commercial muscle rubs.

If you'd like to try capsicum to relieve stomach upset, says Dr. Tyler, try it in small doses—no more than 60 milligrams (just a pinch or two).

"To use capsicum as a muscle rub, mix a little crushed red pepper with rubbing alcohol," he adds. "Keep it out of your eyes, whatever you do. And don't use too much. You could get blisters."

Camomile ● "It's often thought of as an innocuous herb," says Dr. Tyler. "But camomile is an antispasmodic, used extensively throughout Europe for digestive upsets. It has no known toxicity. The only problem is an occasional allergy."

To settle your stomach with camomile, he suggests steeping ½ ounce in 1½ cups of boiling water to make a strong tea. Let it steep ten minutes. Drink it a few times daily, as needed.

Valerian ● Looking for a natural tranquilizer that won't interact with alcohol, as some prescription drugs do? You might try this herb. A small amount — about ¼ teaspoon — in one cup of boiling water is the recommended amount, says Dr. Tyler.

Catnip ● You'd never know it to see what this herb does to your cat, but catnip also appears to be a natural tranquilizer. "Most people who use it make it in a tea, using one to two tablespoons in one cup of boiling water," according to Dr. Tyler.

Hops ● One of the most important ingredients in beer, this herb is also the nutritional equivalent of easy-listening music. "Years ago, it was observed that the people who picked hops became tired and sleepy early in the day," says Dr. Tyler. "No one knew why until it was discovered that hops have mild sedative properties."

You can use hops in a couple of different ways. One way is to sleep on them. "I suggest putting hops in an old muslin pillow and trying it for a good night's rest," says Dr. Tyler. Another way is to make hops tea, using a scant teaspoonful in one cup of boiling water.

Herbs for First Aid and Healthy Arteries

One herb is applied to the skin, and the others are eaten. All three may be beneficial.

Plantain ● Leaves of the spiky weed, commonly found on many lawns, have been widely used over the years to bandage and heal wounds. Its juice has also been used as a remedy for poison ivy. You're supposed to rub the crushed leaves on the affected area, according to Dr. Tyler.

Garlic and Onions ● The claims made on behalf of garlic and onion are numerous, including reports that both these pungent plants reduce the tendency of blood platelets to clot. This may lessen the risk that a clot might block an already narrowed artery, causing heart attack or stroke.

If you use garlic, you should take about one small clove, says Dr. Tyler, and it should be raw. "The more you cook it, the less potent it becomes," he adds. "All the active components of garlic are odoriferous. The deodorized varieties have more or less of the clot-reducing activity removed."

As for onions, Dr. Tyler says, eat as many as you like, preferably raw. Of course, you will soon notice that the one thing onions and garlic cannot do is help you make friends.

A Question of Quality

Suppose you want to try one or more of these herbs. How do you find the right herb for your particular problem? How can you be assured of the product's quality? How do you know, for example, that the feverfew you buy is really feverfew?

It isn't easy. Buying an herbal product is a little like playing Russian roulette, says Dr. Tyler. "Most herbs can be sold, but they can't be labeled with their use." That's because in the United States, herbal preparations are considered food or food additives, such as spices or flavorings—not medicine. You will notice that no therapeutic claims are made for herbs on the package labels.

"In addition, most of the plants are collected in Eastern Europe, Asia and South America, in places where people are not very well educated, where there are very poor quality controls," Dr. Tyler says. "For example, the only 'active' part of camomile is the flower head, not the leaves or stem. But when workers in Argentina go out into the field to pick camomile, they use machines that cut the whole plant. So the camomile you buy might contain leaves and stems, in addition to the flower heads. What we need are standards on these things."

Until then, Dr. Tyler recommends that you buy herbs from a well-known producer who will stand behind the products.

Additionally, you would be wise to follow these words of advice: Get an expert medical diagnosis of your illness before you attempt any treatment, don't pick your own herbs, and use these natural remedies only in moderation.

The Art
of Successful Drinking

Between the teetotalers and the chronic tipplers there exists a group of drinkers who lean on the belief that they have no drinking problem because they display none of the typical signs of alcoholism—a conclusion that's just and accurate for some but possibly misguided for others.

"Most problem drinkers aren't alcoholics; they're moderate drinkers," says Wayne Bartz, Ph.D., a psychologist at American River College, Sacramento, California. Dr. Bartz is also co-author of *The Better Way to Drink,* along with psychologist and alcohol researcher Roger Vogler, Ph.D., of Pomona (California) College. "Many of them think they're normal drinkers, when in fact they may have some abusive drinking habits. But the bad habits can often be corrected before more serious damage is done."

Spotting the unsafe eaters in a crowd is easy—just count paunches. But how do you know if a friend or loved one—or you, for that matter—is an unsafe drinker? It depends on how you define safe and unsafe.

Successful drinkers usually don't drink each day, nor do they drink for more than an hour or so at a time. The amount, which can vary depending on body weight, is usually (for a *large* person) one to four drinks of average size (a 12-ounce beer, 1.25 ounces of liquor or 4 ounces of wine). This usually keeps their blood alcohol (BA) level below or at 0.05, which allows enjoyment of alcohol's beneficial effects but doesn't cause any of the negative physical or psychological consequences associated with drinking too much.

Safe drinkers enjoy social outings with or without alcohol. They never frantically scrounge to find money to buy a drink, and their drinking has never been an issue with friends or family. They have no physical problems caused by alcohol and never miss work because of drinking. They've never been arrested for a drinking-related offense, nor have they developed a tolerance, finding that more and more alcohol is needed to feel the effects. In addition, they don't use alcohol to handle stress or escape from problems.

"No one is perfect, and many successful drinkers become somewhat intoxicated three or four times a year, such as on New Year's Eve, their birthday or some other special occasion," say Dr. Vogler and Dr. Bartz. "But a safe drinker, when intoxicated, won't risk the welfare of others by driving or attempting actions that could harm someone else."

The Unsafe Way

On the other hand, there are the unsafe drinkers, who may or may not drink every day. If they don't drink daily, they tend to overdo it when they do imbibe, and their behavior shows it. Or they may drink moderately on several occasions and then, quite unpredictably, drink far too much the next time. They usually resort to alcohol to help with problems.

Unsafe drinkers tend to rapidly consume straight or strong drinks in gulps, abandoning any intention to limit their intake, whereas safe drinkers retain control by sipping a diluted drink over a longer period of time. Unsafe drinkers may also prefer to socialize only with people who drink, or attend gatherings where there will be alcohol.

Their BA levels can range from 0.05 to 0.20 or higher. (A majority of states regard someone with a BA level of 0.10 as driving under the influence.) "Some unsafe drinkers can hover around the lower end of that scale, but they'll stay there for hours or even days. Others drink faster and rapidly reach high BA levels," says Dr. Vogler.

A person's family history may also suggest the type of drinker he or she may become, because scientists have found that genetics can play a role.

"The theory that some alcohol problems are inherited is widely accepted now," says geneticist James Wilson, Ph.D., head of the University of Colorado-Boulder Institute for Behavioral Genetics. "Now we're searching for a genetic marker to tell us which people are at risk."

Until that time, the best way to find out if someone is

genetically at risk is to sniff around the family tree for hints of alcohol. Geneticists believe a person with an alcoholic father or mother can have a one in four chance of developing similar problems.

"There's no guarantee that a person with a family history of alcoholism will suffer the same fate," adds Dr. Wilson. "If they know they're predisposed to it, however, they might be able to avoid future problems."

Reasons for drinking aside, steps can be taken to either remain a safe drinker or become one. "Establishing and using personal guidelines is like taking out an insurance policy against alcohol abuse," says Dr. Bartz. "It takes very little effort and can actually increase the pleasure of drinking."

First and foremost, know how many drinks someone of your weight can have during the first hour of drinking and remain at or below a BA of 0.05. A 130-pound person may be able to have slightly more than two drinks that hour, a 160-pound person three drinks and a 190-pound person three to four drinks. Regardless of weight, we burn off only about one drink an hour, so any more than one drink per hour after the first hour of drinking will continue to increase the blood alcohol level. Remember that individual metabolisms react differently, and other factors, such as how much food is in the stomach when the drink is consumed, affect the way alcohol is absorbed.

Drink for an hour or less. If you drink for much longer, you'll either consume an unhealthful amount, even though your BA might stay under 0.05, or your BA will exceed 0.05, or both. In any case, the mild pleasantness or "high" that comes with drinking will fade as the BA level exceeds 0.05. If you're going to be at a drinking gathering for several hours, pick an hour during which you will drink alcohol, and consume nonalcoholic beverages the rest of the time.

If you do drink for more than an hour, sip and substitute. If you don't mind missing the "high" many people drink for, spread it out over more time.

When measuring hard liquor, use only a standard 1.25-ounce shot glass and avoid pouring liquor straight from bottle to glass. Watch out for beer. People often think they can drink all they want, but remember that each beer contains slightly more alcohol than a shot of whiskey. Drink only to enhance an already good mood or occasion, not to run from reality. Don't drink while working or performing a distracting task, because your thought may be on your efforts and not the amount of alcohol crossing your lips.

Skip a Day

To avoid becoming alcohol tolerant, don't drink seven days a week. Daily drinkers can unknowingly become tolerant to alcohol and gradually increase intake to realize the feelings they used to experience after a few sips. As a safety net, Dr. Bartz and Dr. Vogler recommend recording consumption for one week every six months. If an increase is noted, stop drinking for a while and figure out why. Safe drinkers avoid alcohol one or more days a week to prevent the body from becoming tolerant.

Never drink and drive. Even though you may feel sober, your driving abilities may be impaired. It's best to make provisions for transportation in advance, such as making sure someone is the "designated driver" who stays sober to do the driving.

Be on guard during high-stress periods. Many people mistakenly believe that alcohol helps solve problems, when actually it hinders. After hitting a BA level of around 0.05, stress relief usually ends and additional alcohol increases anxiety. If you suspect you have a problem, try drinking two less drinks a week until you get to a safe and manageable level of consumption. "Gradual changes are easier than abrupt ones," Dr. Bartz points out. Also shorten your drinking time by starting later and finishing earlier.

Set limits and measure out your daily ration in a separate container so you'll know when the allotment is gone, and each week pour a little less. Also avoid people and places with the potential to send you over your limit. Cut out drinking when it's easy to lose track of consumption, such as during meals.

If alcohol seems to be a problem and none of these suggestions works, professional help is probably in order.

Getting Control
of Your Allergies:
An Expert's Update

From the American College of Allergists

Ah, spring! For most of us, it's a time to kick into high gear. We can't wait to shed our winter layers, sweep the cinders off the walk and bury our noses in a bunch of apple blossoms. Everything's bursting with life.

And that's the problem, at least for those of us with allergies.

Winter puts the freeze on many allergy-causing substances. But come spring, the ground thaws, new grass pushes up, trees sprout leaves, people start working in their yards and ridding their homes of winter's clutter. The result? Air that's thick with mold spores, pollen and dust, inside and out. And the red eyes, runny nose and sneezing that could make you want to spend your summer in hibernation.

That drastic step isn't necessary. Although allergies can't be cured, they can usually be managed very well. The trick is to discover what combination of avoidance, medication and, if necessary, allergy shots will control your symptoms best.

An Overactive Immune System

An allergy is your body's well-meant but misguided attempt to protect you from what it thinks is a hazardous situation. It's an abnormal reaction by your immune system to an ordinarily harmless substance.

"The immune system normally protects the body against harmful invaders, but in allergic people, it reacts to innocuous substances like dust and pollen," says Charles H. Banov, M.D., associate professor of medicine and bacteriology-immunology at the Medical University of South Carolina in Charleston and immediate past president of the American College of Allergists.

Researchers believe that people who develop allergies

114

have a genetic tendency to produce more than normal amounts of a type of antibody (or immunoglobulin) called IgE. The IgE antibody stimulates certain cells to react against allergy-producing particles of dust or pollen. These cells then produce bio-chemicals, such as histamine, that cause sneezing, itching, watery eyes and runny nose.

The medical name for hay fever, or any other short-lived nasal allergy, is seasonal allergic rhinitis (*rhinitis* means "inflammation of the mucous membranes of the nose"). When symptoms are year-round, your condition may be known as perennial allergic rhinitis. Don't let these lengthy names confuse you. They are merely the beginning of a diagnosis.

Unraveling the Mystery

The real clues to your allergies can be found in a complete medical history. "A good allergist asks you a lot of questions first, then does allergy testing," says Michael Kaliner, M.D., chief of the allergic disease section of the National Institute of Allergy and Infectious Diseases, a branch of the National Institutes of Health in Bethesda, Maryland.

"A detailed medical history is more important than any tests," Dr. Kaliner says. "If you screened the entire population with skin tests, 25 to 50 percent would have positive results. But that just means they have antibodies against the material you are testing. It doesn't mean they are symptomatic. An active allergy is diagnosed by medical history, which is then confirmed by skin testing."

For your medical history, you'll be asked not only to identify your symptoms but also to try to remember what age you were when they started, how often they bother you and which months are worst. You'll be asked about allergies in other family members. And you should also be asked about pets, exposure to cigarette smoke, materials in your house, bedding, carpeting, your home's heating system and the kind of work you do.

Even incomplete answers or "best guesses" to some of those questions can provide you and your allergist with a framework from which to proceed.

The Role of Allergy Tests

Your allergist will examine your nose and throat for infection, growths (such as nasal polyps) that might be blocking airways, or malformations (such as a deviated septum). These problems must be ruled out before proceeding.

Allergy tests come next. Although there are now a number of tests available, many allergists still prefer skin-prick testing. In this test, a small amount of an allergen is pushed into the upper layers of the skin of your back or upper arm with a tiny needle. If you're allergic, you react with localized redness, swelling and itching.

"A skin test is safe and painless and provides you with immediate results," Dr. Kaliner says. "It tells you not only if your IgE levels are high but also which allergens are most likely to provoke a reaction. Your doctor can look at the results, recognize whether the reaction is positive or negative, or, if it's in question, decide whether to try a higher concentration of the allergen or go to intradermal testing, which involves injecting the allergen into the deeper layers of the skin."

Some doctors also use a blood test, known as an *in vitro* test and called by many names—RAST, FAST and so forth. With this test, many allergies can be tested with one sample of blood. Its disadvantages are that it's much more expensive and it's less sensitive than skin testing. "It can be useful for people with severe eczema or extremely sensitive skin," Dr. Banov says. "But for most people, it should not substitute for skin testing."

By itself, no blood test or skin-prick test is sufficient to diagnose an allergy. Those tests, along with your history of allergic reactions, are used to help an allergist figure out just what your active allergies are and then to take action.

For any allergy, your first line of defense should be staying out of its way. That might be easy if your allergy is to cats or shrimp. When you are allergic to tree or grass pollen, though, you might wish you could stop breathing for a few weeks. Since you are unable to do that, you could try to stay indoors on dry, breezy days, when pollen counts are at their highest.

Using air conditioning in your house and car during the pollen season can help keep allergens at bay indoors. But be sure you replace the filters once a month.

FOUR SPECIAL TIPS
FOR THE ALLERGIC

Here are some strategies to help you cope with some allergy-aggravating situations.

Making mowing more tolerable. If mowing your lawn leaves you stuffed up, headachy and irritable, perhaps you should be swinging in a hammock instead.

People who develop symptoms when they mow their lawns could be allergic to grass pollen (yes, even low-cut lawns produce pollen, and they also collect pollen from other grasses). But it's thought that they are probably reacting to molds stirred up from the earth by the mower blade.

The best solution is avoidance: Get someone else to mow your lawn, allergy doctors say. If you can't afford that, try wearing a surgical mask to filter out big airborne particles. You might also try taking an antihistamine before mowing, as long as you're confident it won't make you drowsy. If that doesn't work, your doctor may recommend a drug, nasal cromolyn or nasal steroids, that would help all your seasonal allergies.

Of course, you could also buy a goat. Or turn at least part of your lawn into a beautiful natural meadow that seldom needs mowing.

Gardening with less discomfort. If you simply must get out and scratch in your garden come spring, despite your allergies, here are ways to make it easier.

• Wear gloves, especially when you are pulling weeds in your garden. You'll be protected from fuzzy or sticky vegetation that could cause skin reactions.
• Mulch with black plastic rather than straw. Straw contains grass pollens, dust and mold.
• Garden in the evening, when pollen counts are at their lowest, or after a rain.
• Water regularly and thoroughly to keep down dust.
• Be careful not to inhale insecticide powders or sprays, which could aggravate allergies.

Blocking dust. Spring housecleaning can stir huge amounts of household dust into the air. If you're allergic to dust, spend the day having a manicure and massage and let someone else do your dirty work, says Michael

(continued)

**FOUR SPECIAL TIPS
FOR THE ALLERGIC— *Continued***

Kaliner, M.D., chief of the allergic disease section of the National Institute of Allergy and Infectious Diseases, Bethesda, Maryland. If you're determined to tackle it yourself, keep the doors and windows open to let the dust out. Wear a surgical mask and take an antihistamine before cleaning. Where you can, wet-mop rather than vacuum. It's best to keep a relatively sparse house—no deep pile rugs or elaborate curtains.

If dust seems to cause year-long allergy symptoms, consider allergen immunotherapy. Researchers now think the main allergen in dust is a microscopic creature called a dust mite, and it's possible to get injections specifically against mites.

Reducing pollen. Air conditioning helps keep pollens out of your house. And it removes humidity from the air, which usually makes people with allergies feel better.

Make sure you keep the air conditioner's vent closed, so it's not drawing in pollen-laden outside air. Also, research shows that often there is a brief "burst" of mold contamination when an air conditioner is turned on because of mold inside the machine. So turn it on and leave the room for half an hour. This gives any molds in the room time to dissipate.

Keep the temperature as warm as you can tolerate—around 70°F is perfect. Many people, whether they are allergic or not, are bothered by too strong a breeze and temperatures that are set too low.

And you may want to make your bedroom into an allergy-free zone, especially if dust or pets seem to aggravate your symptoms. Discard dust-catching rugs and curtains and encase your mattress in a plastic cover. Make the bedroom off-limits to pets. Consider renting a tabletop air cleaner to remove even more particles. And avoid irritants that can make your allergy symptoms worse—cigarette smoke, aerosol sprays, fragrances and exhaust and paint fumes.

Using Allergy Drugs Safely

Most people can't completely avoid the substances that cause their allergies, so they may turn to medications to control their symptoms.

Antihistamines are the oldest, safest and most widely used allergy drugs. They block the action of histamine and other related biochemicals that can contract air passages or cause sneezing or itching. They're especially useful for treating hay fever.

"Antihistamines have proved to be generally effective, very well tolerated medications," says Dr. Kaliner. Some people can take antihistamines for years with good results. Others find that after a while the drugs don't work as well or that they cannot tolerate the side effects, particularly drowsiness.

"If one of our patients tends to become less responsive to an antihistamine, we would switch him to another," Dr. Kaliner says. (There are six chemically distinct classes of this drug.) "But our experience has been that if you start a patient on a small dose and gradually build up to a full therapeutic dose, you can keep him at that dosage with no problems."

A nonsedating antihistamine was approved by the U.S. Food and Drug Administration in 1984. The drug, chemically known as terfenadine and marketed as Seldane, is available by prescription only. Other nonsedating antihistamines are expected to be approved soon.

Over-the-counter (OTC) antihistamines work well for many people with mild to moderate seasonal allergies, says Harold Nelson, M.D., of the National Jewish Center for Immunology and Respiratory Medicine in Denver.

"Nonprescription antihistamines are a safe, cost-effective way to take care of an allergy problem, particularly if someone needs them only intermittently," Dr. Nelson says. OTCs aren't quite as strong or as long-acting as their prescription counterparts, and there are fewer classes of the drug available. But the most commonly used antihistamine, Chlor-trimeton, is basically the same in both its prescription and nonprescription forms.

Many antihistamine medications, both prescription and OTC, also contain decongestants, drug ingredients that constrict the tiny blood vessels in the nose and thus relieve swelling and stuffiness. "We'll generally try people first on antihistamines alone," Dr. Banov says. "But many of my patients find they need both drugs. And the stimulant effect of decongestants counteracts the antihistamine's sedation."

Dr. Kaliner uses relatively few decongestants for runny noses, sneezing or itching. "When our patients have nasal congestion in addition to [other symptoms] or as their only symptom, we try decongestants, but we're cautious because they can cause unwanted side effects such as nervousness, tremor, rapid heartbeat and raised blood pressure," he says. In older men, decongestants can contribute to urinary retention. Over-the-counter medications are less likely to contain decongestants if they are marketed specifically for allergies, not colds. Check the label.

Taking a nonprescription antihistamine/decongestant during the time your allergy symptoms are at their worst—for instance, the six weeks of ragweed season just before the first frost—is perfectly safe and acceptable, Dr. Nelson says. But you should see an allergist if OTCs don't work for you, if drowsiness or other side effects bother you, or if your allergy symptoms include such signs of asthma as wheezing or a tight chest.

Two major new types of drugs are also available for allergy use, although just how and when they are used depends on the doctor.

Steroids can reduce inflammation in the nose and chest, which makes these drugs very helpful for treating hay fever and asthma, especially when used in combination with antihistamines. Topical steroids are either sprayed into the nose, used as eyedrops or inhaled (for asthma), so they are better targeted to the areas where they are needed. They are also prepared so that any active part of the drug that is absorbed into the bloodstream is readily destroyed in the liver. This avoids the bad side effects of oral and injected steroids.

Dr. Kaliner uses steroid nasal sprays frequently. "They markedly improve the effectiveness of antihistamines and can safely be used even with patients with mild allergies," he says. "They're excellent used in combination with antihistamines and with another allergy drug, nasal cromolyn. Together, they're very effective."

Dr. Banov turns to steroid sprays only when antihistamines, decongestants and allergy shots have failed. "They don't produce as many side effects as oral or injected steroids, but they do sometimes cause local irritation and bleeding in the nose," he says.

Steroids don't begin to work until they've been used for a week to ten days. They must be taken continually during allergy season.

Another new drug, cromolyn sodium, stops cells from releasing histamine. It's the only drug that prevents allergic reactions before they begin. There are now cromolyn preparations to treat each of the three major target organs for allergy and asthma: drops for eyes, spray for nose and inhalant for lungs.

Like topical steroids, cromolyn must be taken continually during the allergy season. "Except for a few rare cases of irritation of the nose, cromolyn probably has the fewest side effects of any nasal medications," Dr. Kaliner says. While it doesn't help everyone, it works best in the most allergic people.

The Addicted Nose

There are several nonprescription medications that most allergists tell their patients to avoid.

People with allergies should be careful using nose drops and sprays. "People's noses get hooked on them, so that they require more and more just to stay open," says Dr. Banov. "We tell people never to use them for more than three days." Weaning someone off nose sprays can be an effort. "If they can't go cold turkey, we'll start them on a nasal steroid," Dr. Banov says. "When that drug has built up enough to be effective, we'll start cutting back the spray. Sometimes, though, people's noses are so clogged up from responding to nose sprays that it's impossible to get an intranasal steroid in. In certain cases we have to initially use oral steroids."

If your seasonal symptoms include asthma, there are things you should know about over-the-counter inhalants. "They are mostly epinephrine (adrenaline), and we can't recommend them," Dr. Kaliner says. "They are very short-acting and have major side effects, such as tremor and rapid heartbeat."

Should You Have Allergy Shots?

If drugs don't do the trick, your doctor may suggest allergy shots, or allergen immunotherapy, as it's called these days.

The principle behind allergen immunotherapy is to inject gradually increasing doses of an allergen over a period of time so the patient gradually builds up resistance to that substance. The shots make the body produce more of a certain kind of "blocking" antibody (called IgG), which can react with an allergy-producing particle before it reaches cells. The shots also eventually produce lower levels of IgE antibodies. Both of these changes make a person less sensitive to allergens.

Immunotherapy is generally a treatment of last resort, says Dr. Nelson. "Allergy shots involve a lot of time and expense and should be reserved for people who can't get adequate relief with simple and safe drug treatment. I like my patients to at least try a medication. If it doesn't work or they don't like the side effects, or if they're someone who just doesn't like to take medicines, then we'll consider shots." Most doctors like their patients to get regular injections for two to three years.

One notable exception to the "drugs first" treatment regimen is asthma. "I'd start allergy injections more readily in someone with asthma," Dr. Nelson says. "A number of studies show that allergic reactions in the lungs make asthmatics much more susceptible to cold air, cigarette smoke and exercise. In a person with asthma, an allergic reaction can produce increased sensitivity to nonallergenic substances for up to two weeks."

Immunotherapy has about an 85 percent success rate in people who have stubborn allergies to grass, ragweed, trees and dust. It also works well against sensitivity to stinging insects, but not against mold allergies.

"Success" in this instance means a significant reduction in allergy symptoms and less need for medication. It doesn't necessarily mean a cure, although some people are totally symptom free after treatment.

And success is directly related to dosage, Dr. Nelson says.

That's important, because, he says, "an appalling number of doctors aren't giving adequate doses of allergens. I'm afraid they are more interested in avoiding reactions than in the efficacy of what they are doing."

The best way to tell if you are getting an adequate dose is if you react to your extracts periodically. You'll have a diffuse area of redness, swelling and itching at the site of the shot, especially as your dosage is increased.

"If you get your injection week after week and never have even a local reaction, you should question whether you are getting adequate treatment," Dr. Nelson says. And if you're on maintenance shots, the extract should be darker in color, not clear.

This is a good reason to be seeing a doctor who is "board-certified," that is, a doctor who has gone through residency training in internal medicine or pediatrics and a two-year training program in allergy and has passed a test given by the American Board of Allergy and Immunology.

Some Opt for Maintenance

Many people who complete a course of immunotherapy and do well at first find their allergies slowly returning, until four or five years later they're right back where they started, Dr. Nelson says. "We see people who have cycled through allergy shots up to three times. They've gone through them, gotten better, gone off and gotten worse."

Some of these people choose to continue their allergy shots indefinitely. "Certainly, once someone is doing well, injections are needed only every six weeks to maintain them at that point," Dr. Nelson says.

Doctors expect to have better weapons in their arsenal against allergy in the next few years, including more effective methods of immunotherapy and new drugs, similar to antihistamines, that neutralize the biochemicals that cause allergy symptoms. They also hope to learn more about how people develop allergies, and find strategies for prevention.

If you need help finding a local doctor with specialized allergy training, write to the American College of Allergists, 800 East Northwest Highway, Suite 101, Mt. Prospect, IL 60056, or call (312) 255-0380.

A New Cholesterol-Buster Comes to Town

Charcoal is catching fire.

Not just any charcoal, and certainly not what you use to grill your chicken and fill the neighbor's backyard with smoke.

It's activated charcoal—wood, nutshells or vegetable matter that is roasted without oxygen until it is glossy black, then ground into fine particles and steamed at very high temperatures to open the pinpoint pores dotting each particle's surface.

Because these pores have been found to latch onto certain fluids and gases, activated charcoal is a natural, all-purpose filter. You'll find it in foot pads to snuff out sneaker odor, for instance. But in a purified form it is also used as an oral antidote for people who've swallowed poison or overdosed on drugs. It can also be taken to control uncomfortable intestinal gas.

Now activated charcoal is being auditioned for a new and potentially heart-saving role: lowering cholesterol. Early results suggest it might be more powerful than conventional drug treatment, with none of the side effects.

A study by scientists in Finland has made charcoal a hot topic among researchers in the United States.

Seven patients in the Finnish study were given about ¼ ounce of activated charcoal three times a day for four weeks. At the end, their blood levels of low-density lipoprotein (LDL) cholesterol—the harmful kind that clogs arteries—had fallen 41 percent. To put these results in perspective, consider that conventional drugs lower LDL by only about 16 percent *(Lancet)*.

At the same time, levels of high-density lipoprotein (HDL) cholesterol rose slightly. HDL is considered a protective factor against heart disease.

Although raising HDL is beneficial, it's also important to reduce cholesterol levels overall. High levels of total cholesterol have been linked with increased risk of heart disease.

Charcoal's Magnetic Personality

To Eli A. Friedman, M.D., a medical researcher at the State University of New York Health Science Center in Brooklyn, these findings strongly indicate a need to investigate activated charcoal further.

"The key question is its efficiency," he says. "Will it work in more than seven people?"

On the basis of the Finnish study and previous research of his own, Dr. Friedman suspects charcoal may lower cholesterol by binding, or clinging to it. Here's how.

Picture the surface of a grain of activated charcoal as something like the face of a microscopic moon, with craters of many sizes, from small to large. Scientists have long known that molecules of certain substances—intestinal gas or poison, for example—are attracted to these holes.

When molecules want to move in, a bit of charcoal can be very accommodating. Because each grain has pores of many different sizes and shapes, it gives molecules of varying sizes and shapes places to roost. A hefty molecule of cholesterol might slip into one cranny, while a much smaller molecule of intestinal gas would fit into another.

One of the advantages of activated charcoal is that the body doesn't absorb it from the intestine. Charcoal simply picks up molecules, like passengers on a bus, and heads for the nearest exit ramp out of the body. That's what makes charcoal so safe.

If charcoal can safely ferry excess cholesterol out of the body over the course of your lifetime, so much the better. Over time, cholesterol and fat deposits can block the passage of blood through the coronary arteries, possibly triggering a heart attack or stroke. That hardening of the arteries is called atherosclerosis.

New Hope for Kidney Patients

But for some people, lowering cholesterol is not just a long-term strategy. It is an immediate concern.

People with kidney disease, for example, are quite vulnerable to increased blood fat and an increase of atherosclerosis. In fact, atherosclerosis is one of the leading causes of death among long-term dialysis patients because of the abnormal lipid metabolism of failing kidneys.

Previous research by Dr. Friedman and his associates

addressed the kidney patient's urgent concerns about atherosclerosis. Aware of charcoal's stick-to-itiveness, Dr. Friedman tried using charcoal to lower harmful blood fats.

"We were looking for a way to lower blood fat levels without hurting the person," recalls Dr. Friedman. "We knew that charcoal was cheaper and probably safer than drugs."

In Dr. Friedman's study, six patients took 35 grams of charcoal—a little over an ounce—every day. At the end of 24 weeks, cholesterol levels had dropped as much as 43 percent. Levels of triglycerides, another blood fat, fell as much as 76 percent.

Although the study didn't differentiate between LDL and HDL, the findings were significant, since overall cholesterol levels in many patients dropped, particularly among those with the highest cholesterol.

Cholesterol reduction is particularly important for those at immediate risk, like kidney patients, but it's also a priority for the rest of us.

According to nationwide studies, more than half of all adult men have cholesterol levels high enough to put them at risk for heart attack. Dietary changes—such as reducing intake of saturated fat and cholesterol—will go a long way toward reducing that risk for those of us who don't yet have heart disease.

But according to the Finnish researchers, more needs to be done for people who already have dangerously high cholesterol levels. The results of their study of activated charcoal, they conclude, suggest this harmless and potentially helpful substance is an avenue of research clearly worth pursuing.

Less Noise for More Health

A good theme song for America right now would not be "Sounds of Silence." Progress has made our lives easier but certainly not quieter. The clamor has in large part been responsible for making impaired hearing a problem for an estimated one out of eight Americans. More chronic disability is due to bad hearing right now than to bad backs!

But eardrums aren't all that's taking a beating. Studies suggest that the racket of modern life may be raising our blood pressure, increasing our risk of heart disease, chipping away at our mental stability, giving us ulcers and possibly even souring our personalities. In one experiment, researchers found that people were less likely to help someone pick up books when there was a lawn mower running nearby.

"Noise is a more hazardous pollutant than many of us realize," says Arline L. Bronzaft, Ph.D., chairperson of the Noise Committee of the Council on the Environment of New York City and professor of psychology at Lehman College in Brooklyn. "Some studies suggest it may even make a dent in the human sex drive."

Good grief.

"Much can be done to control noise, however, and that's the message we've got to get across," Dr. Bronzaft says. "People can control noise because people are the ones who make noise."

More Quiet on the Home Front

And perhaps the best place for most of us to start turning down the volume is right in our own homes. "You may not be able to control the trucks that roar past your house, but you can control the appliances you use and how loud you play the TV and the stereo. People don't often realize it, but the amount of background noise they live with can be aggravating on a semi-conscious level."

We hear you, Dr. Bronzaft. The average blender makes as much noise as the average subway. Most vacuum cleaners put out as many decibels as rush-hour traffic. Start adding up the clamor of these appliances, and you can have bedlam on your hands.

Worse yet can be the volume "wars" that can develop: Valerie turns up her stereo to drown out Jennifer's TV, which is turned up to drown out Dad in the basement playing handyman with his table saw. The escalation can lead to decibel levels far in excess of what's considered safe for the human ear. And that's before family members all start shouting at each other to turn down respective noisemakers!

YOUR LIFE IS TOO LOUD IF . . .

The experts agree that exposure to noise levels in excess of 85 decibels for eight or more hours a day can eventually harm hearing. Exposure to 115 decibels even for just 15 minutes a day can do the same.

So you do the arithmetic. If the noise in your life is adding up to those levels or higher, you should take definite steps to quiet things down. And remember: Noises compound one another. A stereo in addition to an air conditioner is louder than either alone. Add Junior learning to play the electric guitar and you're talking an ill-advised concert for sure.

Sound	Decibel Level
Refrigerator	50
Ordinary human speech	60
TV or stereo at normal volume	65
Window air conditioner	60-75
Blender	65-85
Noisy restaurant	70-75
Vacuum cleaner	70-80
Electric shaver	75
Busy traffic	75-85
Alarm clock	80
Subway train	80-105
Screaming child	90-115
Live rock music	90-130
Jackhammer	100
Chain saw	100
Motorcycle	100
Automobile horn	110
Loud thunder	120
Jet engine at takeoff	120-140
Air-raid siren	140
Rocket taking off	180

"Your home should be your haven—especially if you have to put up with a lot of noise at work or while commuting," Dr. Bronzaft says. "Studies show that the effects of noise on the human ear are cumulative—extended exposures to moderately loud situations, in other words, can be more damaging than shorter exposures to noise that may be considered extreme."

With that in mind, here are some tips for muffling the home front.

● Try not to use more than one noisy appliance at a time. Blenders, vacuum cleaners, dishwashers, garbage disposals and hair dryers are the noisiest. Also try to keep appliances in good working order.

● Use earphones to prevent volume wars. If Valerie wants to listen to music and Jennifer's in the mood for TV, put Valerie in earphones.

● Encourage noisy hobbyists to hobby outside. If that's not possible or if outdoor noise would bother neighbors, maybe the hobbyist can have his work area soundproofed. Many effective insulating products for walls, ceilings and floors are available.

● Take time for a silence break. Many families become so accustomed to their domestic ruckus that they lose sight of how quiet things could be, Dr. Bronzaft says. To prevent this, try imposing periods of total silence from time to time, as a way of reminding yourselves of just what an uproar you put up with.

● Realize that plush furnishings can do ears a favor. They absorb sound rather than bouncing it back into the environment.

More Peace at Work

Quieting things at work can be more difficult, because you're not in control, but by no means does that mean the situation is hopeless. "There are ear protectors of all shapes and sizes, and they work," Dr. Bronzaft says.

Seconding that opinion is hearing-conservation specialist Donald C. Gasaway, who explains that ear protectors actually help rather than hinder workers from hearing the sounds they need to hear in order to work safely. "Hearing protectors function much as sunglasses do—they filter out the 'glare' of loud noise and by doing so enhance the ability to hear desired signals. Workers can actually hear better in noise if they wear hearing protection."

Carrying the sunglass analogy one step further, however, Gasaway explains that wearing hearing protection unnecessarily is like wearing sunglasses in the dark: The ability to hear sounds important for safety could be impaired. As a rule of thumb, if you must raise your voice to communicate at a distance of one foot or if you must shout to be heard at a distance of three feet, then hearing protection is necessary. Otherwise it's overkill, Gasaway says.

And what about listening to music through earphones as a way of escaping unpleasant racket?

It's probably not a good idea, Gasaway says, because you're really only adding to your noise level, not diminishing it. That can be bad for your safety as well as your hearing, since you're making yourself even more oblivious to your surroundings.

Niacin: A Happy Surprise for the Heart

It's highly unusual for researchers to discover impressive new benefits of a medical treatment years after a study has ended and the medications given during that time have been stopped. But that's what scientists at a Maryland research institute found recently.

The researchers were doing a follow-up to the well-known Coronary Drug Project. That study, which ended in 1975, was a huge, six-year-long nationwide trial of five potential treatments for heart disease. Sponsored by the National Heart, Lung and Blood Institute, Bethesda, Maryland, and run by top researchers around the country, it enrolled 8,341 patients, all with coronary artery disease.

The initial results of the study were fairly impressive but a little difficult to interpret. They showed that people who daily took three grams (3,000 milligrams) of niacin, a B-complex vitamin, had about 27 percent fewer nonfatal heart attacks than people taking other drugs or a nontherapeutic placebo. (When used in such large doses, niacin is generally referred to as a drug rather than a nutrient.) But the results didn't show a drop in the rate of *fatal* heart attacks in the people taking niacin.

"We didn't really play up the benefits of niacin at that time because it hadn't shown a decrease in mortality," says Paul Canner, Ph.D., of the Maryland Medical Research Institute in Baltimore, one of the study's researchers. "We felt that if it wasn't helping people live longer, there wasn't much reason to publicize it."

It was a different story for niacin, though, when it came to the recent follow-up of the study's participants.

The group that had been taking the vitamin was now found to have from 9 to 13 percent fewer deaths—from heart disease or from any other cause—than the other groups, including those treated with a still-popular cholesterol-lowering drug clofibrate.

"We were very surprised by this finding," Dr. Canner says. "What surprised me most was how many years later this effect appeared. I never thought it would take this long for additional benefits to show up, or that there would even *be* benefits from niacin this much later."

The Coronary Drug Project isn't the only study to confirm niacin's talent at combating heart disease. In a landmark study published in 1981, researchers at the University of California, San Francisco, tried out a niacin regimen on patients with familial hypercholesterolemia.

People with this condition have a genetic tendency toward superhigh blood cholesterol levels—350 milligrams or more—and used to be consigned to an early death from heart disease.

The San Francisco researchers used a combination of up to 7.5 grams daily of niacin, a drug called colestipol (which binds bile acids and increases the breakdown of cholesterol in the liver) and a diet low in cholesterol and saturated fat. The regimen brought these patients' cholesterol levels back to normal, lowering them by an average of 45 percent.

"This was the first study to show that a drug regimen could normalize the dangerously high blood cholesterol levels in these people," says John Kane, M.D., the study's main researcher. It also showed that niacin and colestipol could act as partners against the ravages of heart disease. These two drugs are now a standard treatment for people with familial hypercholesterolemia.

During his study, Dr. Kane noted that fatty deposits found

on the tendons of his patients shrank as their cholesterol levels dropped. "It's encouraging that this regimen removed cholesterol from a tissue site," Dr. Kane says. "While these deposits aren't exactly the same as the fatty plaques found in the arteries, there is some inference from this that you might be reversing the actual lesions in the arteries."

Another study published by a group headed by lipid researcher Scott Grundy, M.D., now at the University of Texas Health Science Center, Dallas, gave yet more credence to niacin's benefits.

This study included 12 patients who were considered typically at risk for having a heart attack. They had high cholesterol and triglyceride levels. Some showed signs of clogged arteries. Patients took one gram of niacin three times a day for one month. At the end of that time, their cholesterol levels had dropped an average of 22 percent and their triglycerides had dropped 52 percent *(Journal of Lipid Research)*.

"Niacin, when taken in large doses, works by decreasing the liver's production of harmful blood fats," says Cara East, M.D., a specialist in lipid metabolism at the University of Texas Health Science Center. "It is the only drug that clearly works that way, and it's the only drug that is clearly effective at lowering both triglycerides and cholesterol. So, in that sense, it has an advantage over any other drug."

Downs LDL, Ups HDL

Niacin hits especially hard on low-density and very low-density lipoproteins (LDL and VLDL), both artery-clogging blood fats. At the same time, it raises the levels of high-density lipoproteins (HDL), which help protect against heart disease.

As a result of both these actions, niacin has a strong effect on the ratio of total cholesterol to HDL. And that ratio may be the most sensitive indicator yet of somone's chances for heart disease, says James Alderman, M.D., a Framingham, Massachusetts, cardiologist and Beth Israel Hospital/Harvard Medical School researcher.

"In lipid research trials using diet alone or drugs other than niacin, it's been clearly shown that improving the ratio of total cholesterol to HDL can decrease mortality from coronary artery disease," Dr. Alderman says.

"When you compare the lipid profiles—the complete analysis of blood fats—of patients from these trials with patients taking niacin, it becomes apparent that the niacin is creating more favorable changes in the ratio of total cholesterol to HDL, which hopefully will translate into fewer heart attacks and longer life."

Dr. Alderman recently completed a pilot study of niacin, using amounts smaller than those used in previous studies. "We decided to try a lower total dose, because previous studies using high doses reported a high incidence of mild but unpleasant side effects," he says. "Our goal was to get our heart patients up to two grams a day." The patients who reached that goal, about half the group of 101, showed significant improvements in blood fats. Their HDL levels, in particular, increased dramatically.

"A ratio of total cholesterol to HDL greater than 5 places a person at higher risk for coronary heart disease," Dr. Alderman says. "In patients in our study, the total cholesterol-to-HDL ratio fell from 7.1 to 4.8." Among the patients taking one gram or less of niacin, the average ratio fell from 7.4 to 5.6. And in those patients taking more than one gram of niacin per day, the ratio fell from 6.9 to 4.4.

"The benefits were dose related," Dr. Alderman says. "In general, the more niacin a person could take, the better the results."

Sidestepping Side Effects

Tolerance has traditionally been a problem with niacin. Common side effects are flushing, itching and stomach upset. But researchers now have a number of ways to avoid these problems. They place their patients on gradually increasing dosages, starting with 100 milligrams twice a day the first week and working up to several thousand milligrams daily over the course of a month or more. If side effects such as flushing do occur, one regular aspirin a day controls the symptoms for many people. For others, time-release niacin does the trick, but it is not as well absorbed and therefore may be less effective.

There is no proof that small amounts of niacin—100 milligrams or less a day—could help to prevent heart disease. "Our patients taking smaller amounts of niacin were still tak-

---

KNOW YOUR NIACIN

Niacin and related compounds have sometimes been labeled interchangeably, so there may be some confusion about what form you are using.

Only one form of niacin has a cholesterol-lowering effect. That form is referred to as "niacin" or "nicotinic acid." Niacinamide, a B-complex form that is popular because it does not cause flushing, has no effect on blood lipids.

---

ing an average of 700 milligrams a day," Dr. Alderman says. That's still many times more than the Recommended Dietary Allowance of 18 milligrams for an adult male. Even the richest source of niacin, beef liver, has only 4.3 milligrams per ounce.

Researchers emphasize that the use of large amounts of niacin does need to be medically supervised. Niacin in such large doses can cause some changes in liver function, requiring testing by a physician. These changes can be controlled under medical supervision, Dr. Alderman says.

Niacin can also raise blood glucose levels, so its use should be carefully monitored in diabetics. Because it has an effect on uric acid levels, niacin can potentially aggravate gout.

"Niacin certainly shows a tremendous amount of promise, though further large-scale testing is needed to confirm the results of our pilot study," Dr. Alderman says. "Our patients showed great improvement in their lipid profiles and they tolerated the niacin well. So hopefully they could remain on long-term therapy with this medication. I find niacin a very acceptable therapy, one that could turn out to have significant long-term results. Hopefully niacin will someday prove effective as part of any program for heart disease."

The Health Power of Perfect Sleep

From the Association of Sleep Disorders Centers

All right, stop nodding off and pay attention.

Yes, *you.* You with the I-haven't-slept-well-since-1974 look on your face. You with the droopy eyes and the slurred speech and the zombie walk. Keep your lids propped open for just ten minutes while you read this chapter. It has good news for you.

The science of sleep is in its heyday, offering practical solutions to sleep problems you may have thought were hopeless.

Nowadays, for mild insomnia, life-threatening sleep apnea (a condition in which breathing difficulties cause interrupted sleep) and anything in between, there's usually an effective treatment or simple preventive. And contrary to sleep mythology, you can often solve sleep problems without sleeping pills or long-term sleep therapy.

Because of advances in sleep research in the past 15 years, sleep experts (they're called somnologists) have been able to help people who haven't had a decent night's sleep in 30 years, who can't adjust to shift work, or who can't get to sleep or stay asleep or stay awake during the day. They've pinpointed the steps that most people should take to help assure themselves that they get a good night's sleep. Sleep experts have identified 120 sleep or arousal disorders, tracked the dark physiological processes of slumber and developed high-tech methods for diagnosing sleep glitches that used to be the body's own secret.

So here's a review of what the experts have learned and how it can help you embrace sweet sleep.

The Mechanisms of Sleep

ZZZZZZZZ . . . For Dagwood, Andy Capp and other comic-strip nappers, this is the shorthand for sleep. The body stops, the eyes close and Z's pop into the word balloons to symbolize that nothing much is going on.

Similar to real sleep, right? The brain switches off, everything else downshifts to automatic pilot and . . . ZZZZZZZZ.

Wrong, all wrong. Somnologists now know that sleep isn't simple, passive or uniform. In slumber, all kinds of things happen in complex rhythms and cycles—things that may have a profound effect on the wide-awake you.

Among the goings-on are two physiological patterns or states called rapid eye movement (REM) sleep and nonrapid eye movement (NREM) sleep. In REM sleep your eyes dart about beneath closed eyelids. You're likely to dream, yet your brain waves are like those during wakefulness. And you're almost completely paralyzed—certain muscle groups actually shut down. If you're male, you'll probably have an erection (even babies do); if you're female, vaginal excitation may occur.

NREM sleep differs from REM sleep in a lot more ways than just eye movements. It progresses through four stages, from semiwakefulness to deep sleep, where brain waves are big and slow (called delta waves) and you're difficult to rouse. In NREM sleep you can move about, and dreams are likely to be few and far between. In the last two stages of NREM your body secretes big doses of growth hormone—which is why sleep experts think these stages are somehow "restorative" for the body.

At bedtime NREM sleep comes first; it lasts about 90 minutes. Then REM sleep occurs, usually lasting about 5 minutes. Then this NREM/REM cycle repeats (about five times in eight hours of sleep), with NREM getting gradually shorter and REM getting longer—a slow, silent roller-coaster ride in the night.

Overlaid on these cycles (what somnologists call "sleep architecture") are other physiological patterns. Body temperature, blood pressure, heart rate, breathing and metabolic rate all change during sleep.

Unexpected Results of Poor Sleep

And because sleep is filled with so many rhythms and changes, because it's not comic-strip simple, it can affect your health in unexpected ways.

For example, some illnesses that are present during waking hours may get worse in sleep. The bodily machinations of slumber can aggravate emphysema, chronic bronchitis, asthma, cluster headaches, heart disease, ulcers and more.

And now it's clear that some diseases and life-threatening situations show up *only* during sleep. Merrill M. Mitler, Ph.D., sleep expert and secretary/treasurer of the Association of Sleep Disorders Centers, says, "It's possible for someone to appear to be perfectly healthy during the day but be literally near death during sleep. Sleep apnea is the most notable example of this, but there are other serious disorders that simply may not exist in the wakeful state. These are problems we can detect in sleep disorders centers."

Insomniacs "don't get no respect." At least it seems that way most of the time. If you've endured a restless night, who wants to hear about it? Your mother, maybe. Who wants to joke about it? Everyone. And why not? It's not as though insomnia is a symptom of anything, is it?

Among sleep doctors, insomnia is no joke. It's a caution light. It is indeed by definition a symptom: Something's amiss. Perhaps something minor, major or in between, but something. And it affects you round the clock, not just while you're lying in bed staring at the ceiling.

And it's going around. At any given time, as many as 120 million people may suffer from so-called transient insomnia, the kind that lasts less than three weeks and is caused by things like stress, jet lag, the death of a loved one or loss of a job. Then there are an additional 20 million victims who endure chronic insomnia: long-term poor sleep caused by physical or behavioral problems. Whether you call them transient or chronic, all these insomniacs take too long to fall asleep (generally 30 minutes or more), have trouble staying asleep (awaken too many times or too early) or experience sleep that's too light.

How Do You Know If You Have Insomnia?

Okay, so you don't drop into oblivion as soon as your head hits the pillow, and you're a little fatigued throughout the day—does this mean you're one of these 140 million poor sleepers? And how much sleep is enough sleep to avoid the label of insomniac?

"The best measure of whether you have insomnia is how

you feel during your waking hours," says insomnia expert Milton K. Erman, M.D., of the Sleep Disorders Center at the Scripps Clinic in La Jolla, California. "If you feel alert and you don't nod off during the day even when you're bored stiff, you're probably getting enough good-quality sleep."

Besides, the idea that everyone must get eight hours of shut-eye every night is a myth. True, the average amount of sleep for adults is seven to eight hours, but the range of sleep requirements is vast—about six to nine hours for 90 percent of the population. A few people may need only five hours of sleep or as much as ten.

Confusion about real sleep requirements has even forced some people into a kind of false insomnia: You think you must get eight hours of sleep each night, yet your body really needs only six, so you fret about taking so long to fall asleep or waking up so early.

"Each person has a genetically determined sleep requirement," Dr. Mitler says. "As far as we know, this need doesn't change during adulthood and can't be reduced by 'practice.' The notion that the elderly need less sleep is probably based on the fact that they often get less sleep because of medical problems."

Measure Your Own Sleep Requirement

If you don't know what your sleep requirement is, try this: For one month get the same amount of sleep each night, retiring and rising at precisely the same time. Assess how you feel on this schedule. Then for two weeks, get 30 minutes more or less sleep per night and see if you feel better or worse during the day. Keep up this kind of trial and error until you pin down your RSA (Recommended Snooze Allowance).

So why do so many people fail to meet their sleep quotas or seem not to be refreshed by the sleep they do get? Here are some of the most important insomnia instigators and how to deal with them.

The Effects of Mind Games

The most common causes of insomnia have more to do with your head than dripping faucets or noisy neighbors.

Depression, anxiety, stress, tension, psychoses—these force people to sleep disorders centers in droves.

They're also frequently more manageable than many people think. Severe depression and other serious psychological problems require and often respond to professional help. Mild stress and anxiety usually ease up with relaxation techniques, regular exercise or biofeedback. And certain behavioral sleep-stoppers disappear with regular doses of behavioral counter-measures.

A stressful day, for example, makes it tough for you to fall asleep. So you try harder. And the harder you try, the more uptight you get, becoming more wide-eyed by the hour. So you stop trying—and as you switch on the TV to watch the 4:00 A.M. farm news, you doze off.

The moral: You can't force sleep. So do the opposite, say sleep experts. When you can't drift off, get out of bed and get your mind off sleep. Read, watch TV, knit. And when you finally feel sleepy, return to bed. The next day, rise at your standard time, no matter how late you stayed up, and avoid daytime naps unless they're part of your usual routine. Otherwise, you may end up reversing your body's sleep/wake schedule, sleeping in and retiring later and later.

Then there's this behavioral mixup: Your darkened bedroom, your comfy pillow, your bedtime rituals of brushing your teeth or reading a dull book don't trigger sleep as they do in many people—they stir you up, actually keep you from sleeping. But when you're on the sofa, or when you skip your usual bedtime routine (while traveling, for instance), you can doze off in nothing flat. What's wrong?

Psychologists call it maladaptive conditioning. If your bedroom and bedtime are a pressure cooker where the frustrations of insomnia or daily stress heat up, you can begin to associate them with those frustrations. Pretty soon, everything that should be connected with sleep keeps you wide awake. Often you can get into this odd predicament by doing everything in the world in bed except sleeping—talking on the phone, working, writing letters, paying bills, worrying about tomorrow, eating, watching TV or simply lying in bed fretting about your lack of sleep.

You get out of this mess by breaking the sleep-stopping connections and forming better ones. You start by using your bed *only* for sleep and sex, and by going to bed only when you're really sleepy. If you hop into bed and then start to feel restless, use the nonforced-sleep technique mentioned above, even if it means getting out of bed a dozen times.

During the first night of this new conditioning, you probably won't sleep much, but any loss of shut-eye will help you sleep better the next night. By the third night, you'll probably drop off to dreamland on the first or second try.

Night Moves

You fall asleep and soon a strange thing happens: Your legs begin to twitch about every 30 to 50 seconds for up to an hour, then stop, then start again for another staccato round. The barrages continue throughout the night, rousing you slightly at every twitch, maybe hundreds of times. In the morning you remember little or nothing of this torment (though your bed partner may complain plenty about your kicking), but you may feel as though you hardly slept.

This affliction is periodic leg movements (technically, nocturnal myoclonus), a major type of insomnia, particularly in the elderly. It's not the same thing as restless legs syndrome, the annoying sensation in the legs that compels people to move them, sometimes keeping them from falling asleep. And it shouldn't be confused with so-called hypnic jerks, the normal twitches that may ignite in certain muscles just as we drift off to sleep.

It happens more often in women than in men and seems to get worse with age and after pregnancy or back injury.

"The cause of periodic leg movements is unknown," says somnologist Stuart J. Menn, M.D., a Scripps Clinic expert on the medical causes of insomnia. "Often its effect is that it prevents sleep from getting down to the deeper NREM levels, so the patient may feel that his sleep is not very refreshing or restorative, that he's fatigued or drowsy during the day."

Standard treatment is a prescription drug called clonazepam, which doesn't banish the twitches entirely but reduces their number or makes them less likely to disturb sleep. It improves sleep in two-thirds of the people who take it. Not-so-standard treatments (with a less impressive track record) are regular exercise during the day and relaxation techniques before bedtime.

How Drugs Can Help or Hurt

Everybody knows that too much caffeine too close to bedtime can make it tough for you to fall asleep. Fewer know that it can actually wake you, because caffeine's stimulant effect may not kick in until hours after you consume it. But you may be surprised to learn the truth about some other chemicals and their effect on sleep.

Surprise: A little drink before bedtime is not the great sleep enhancer it's cracked up to be. Yes, a nightcap may relax you so you fall asleep more easily, but the sedative effects may last only four to five hours and leave you awake and hung over at 4:00 A.M. Another problem is that alcohol suppresses REM sleep. After this effect wears off, there's a big surge of REM, enough to wake you up fretting, with your head full of dreams.

Surprise: Smoking doesn't relax you so you can sleep better—it disrupts sleep. After all, it is a stimulant.

Surprise: Sleeping pills are often a major factor in disturbed sleep. It's not that they don't work. They do. (In fact, today's prescribed sleeping pills are generally safer and more effective than they used to be.) The problem is that they don't work as well as people want them to. When you take them several nights in a row, they may at first do a good job of inducing sleep. But your body builds up tolerance fast, the pills quickly lose their effect and, some sleep experts say, their chronic use makes your insomnia worse. Increasing the dose just escalates the problem. And if you stop taking the pills, you may suffer "rebound insomnia"—your sleeplessness may be worse than ever. Time to get thee to a physician or sleep clinic. (Of course, the sternest warnings about taking sleeping pills go to the people who could be hurt the most by them: the elderly, people with liver and kidney disease, pregnant and lactating women and loud snorers, who are more likely to have breathing disorders.)

Is it ever smart to fight insomnia with sleeping pills?

Sometimes, say somnologists. "Sleeping pills can be useful if used properly," Dr. Erman points out. "In transient insomnia, when we've ruled out serious health problems and when nondrug techniques alone aren't appropriate, we may prescribe sleeping pills for occasional short-term use—for example, for one or two sleepless nights a month. It's the night-after-night downing of sleeping pills that makes matters worse."

And what of other drugs—can they also undo sleep? Some can, like steroids, thyroid preparations and respiratory stimulants for the treatment of lung diseases.

"If you suspect that your medication is disturbing your sleep," Dr. Menn says, "don't stop taking it. Tell your doctor. He may be able to solve the problem by altering the dosage or by substituting another drug."

Stroke-Prevention Surgery: How Safe Is It?

Take your hand and feel the pulse in your neck. That artery, the carotid, is your main lifeline. Your life depends on an adequate supply of the oxygen in your blood getting through this artery to your brain from minute to minute.

A doctor could put a stethoscope to your neck and tell you whether the artery is becoming clogged with fatty buildup due to atherosclerosis. He would hear a bruit (pronounced *brew-ee*)—the sound of blood rushing through a narrowed artery. You may not feel ill, but a bruit signals that something's wrong. If you have a bruit, your chances of having a stroke almost double.

An operation called a carotid endarterectomy opens up and cleans out the carotid artery. It has become the most widely performed noncardiac vascular surgery in the United States, and its popularity is increasing rapidly.

But while most doctors believe that carotid endarterectomies help prevent strokes, researchers are now finding that those who have bruits but no other warning signs of stroke may be better off without the operation.

Recently, researchers at the Cincinnati College of Medicine looked at the results of 1,181 carotid endarterectomies performed over the course of a year. They found the stroke and death rate associated with the procedure "alarming" and expressed concern that carotid endarterectomies are being performed too frequently.

Of the asymptomatic people (those with only bruits but no other real symptoms), 5.3 percent either had a stroke or died during surgery or shortly afterward.

Since half of all endarterectomies are being performed on asymptomatic people, that means there may be approximately 1,000 unnecessary deaths and about 2,000 unnecessary strokes this year as a result of the surgery.

The Cincinnati researchers are not sure whether the procedure is any better than treating patients with aspirin or other drugs. They do suggest, however, that for asymptomatic patients, "a more conservative approach is warranted" until further evidence supports its therapeutic value *(Journal of the American Medical Association).*

"The purpose of our study was to find out what was actually being achieved today in a representative metropolitan community. Then we can focus our decision-making in a more realistic light," says one of the researchers, Richard F. Kempczinski, M.D., a vascular surgeon at the University of Cincinnati College of Medicine.

"As I review the literature and the studies to date, it seems to me that asymptomatic patients are at greater risk because of the surgery than if they didn't have it. But not everyone interprets this the same way," says Mark Dyken, M.D., professor and chairman of the Department of Neurology at the Indiana School of Medicine, Indianapolis, and chairman of the American Heart Association's Stroke Council. "There are a lot of people over age 50 who have varying degrees of atherosclerosis. We know that disease is a risk for stroke, but all the evidence we have is that it's a random risk. It's not directly or closely related to the vessels involved in surgery."

How Strokes Develop

Atherosclerosis is the instigator behind most strokes. The linings of the arteries become thickened by deposits of fat, cholesterol, fibrin (a clotting material), dead cells and calcium. Blood flows through the arteries and veins but tends to clot when it comes in contact with this "garbage," which is politely called plaque. The plaque may be marked with little craters, which can give rise to clots. A blood clot or a piece of the plaque may break off and travel to the brain, causing a stroke.

When that happens, the brain is deprived of oxygen and part of the brain may die. Depending on where the damage occurs, you may develop paralysis, loss of speech, hearing and sight or impairment of the ability to swallow. Usually when these functions are gone, they're gone for good.

The carotid arteries are prime targets for blockages because atherosclerotic buildup occurs most often where vessels narrow and branch off. In your neck, you have two carotids—one on each side—each of which divides into two more arteries: the external carotid and the internal carotid. The external carotids branch off to your head and neck; the internal carotids shoot up to the brain, the optic nerve and retina, passing onto and through a traffic circle in the base of the skull. Both carotids contribute to this circle, which works as a communicating system so that if one artery is blocked, the others may help out.

Before surgery, DIVA (digital intravenous angiography) is performed. This test may have some risks because it involves injecting dye into a vein, but it is highly accurate. An image is created from x-rays taken at different times and stored on a computer. These images combined give an even clearer picture of the extent of the blockage, and surgeons use it like a road map.

During the operation, the carotid artery is opened and the plaque is carefully scraped out. Some surgeons may prefer to use local anesthesia so the patient can report numbness or weakness when the carotid is clamped. Others prefer general anesthesia.

Does Anyone Benefit?

In light of these new findings, who would still benefit from a carotid endarterectomy?

"This is where you come into a gray area," says Howard C. Baron, M.D., attending vascular surgeon at Cabrini Medical

Center and a practicing vascular surgeon in New York. "I feel that if there is a bruit in each artery, this is dangerous, and that person should be operated on. Not simultaneously, but in stages over a period of time. If, in any asymptomatic patient, you find a bruit on only one side that occupies more than 50 percent of the diameter of the internal carotid, that patient is a candidate for surgery and should go through usual diagnostic procedures. If you don't operate, two to five years from now the person may have other systemic diseases, and he becomes a poorer surgical risk."

Other doctors feel strongly that the consequences of the surgery are more dangerous than the operation. "I don't have any of my asymptomatic patients operated on," says Dr. Dyken.

The proper studies haven't been done to find out who is better off with the operation, with medical treatment or with no treatment. Several studies are being proposed for funding and, if they get the go-ahead, a more definitive answer may be available several years down the road. "In the meantime, I think we have to be conservative," Dr. Dyken stresses.

The answer would differ, however, for patients who have symptoms and who have not been helped by medical therapy. "It seems logical to me that if you have a surgeon who has a very low complication rate, those people would be candidates for surgery," adds Dr. Dyken.

Symptoms of Artery Blockage

Symptoms, often produced by episodes called transient ischemic attacks (TIAs), include feelings of numbness or weakness in the face, arm or leg on one side, difficulty speaking, memory lapses or temporary blindness. The blindness, which usually affects just one eye, has been described by patients as having a curtain pulled down over their eye. The sight gradually clears. They may also have dizziness or double vision or stagger while walking.

TIAs usually last from 30 seconds to 3 minutes. Almost all clear within 30 minutes. A person may have only a few attacks or several hundred. A stroke may occur after only one or two attacks or after a hundred have occurred over a period of weeks or months. Sometimes the attacks gradually cease.

If surgery is the appropriate choice, patients should ask a

neurologist in their area for the name of a good surgeon who is getting excellent results with carotid endarterectomies, Dr. Kempczinski suggests. In addition, a list of doctors in your area who specialize in this type of surgery may be obtained from your local medical society. And don't hesitate to ask several doctors and patients for recommendations.

When surgery is not called for, there are several alternatives. Some blockages in the carotid may just be checked periodically, and others can be treated medically with anticlotting drugs or aspirin to keep the blood flowing freely.

Many researchers think that the death rate from stroke has declined in recent years because high blood pressure is now being controlled more effectively. High blood pressure, in fact, is one of the greatest risk factors for stroke. You may also reduce your risk of having a stroke by controlling diabetes, eating a low-fat diet, exercising regularly, not drinking excessively and not smoking.

Weight-Loss and Fitness Updates

Walk Off Your Hips and Wake Up Your Health!

If you ever find yourself at the grocery store standing in line behind Gary Yanker, an author and walking expert who's logged more miles on foot than many people have traveled by car, get him to tell you about a conversation he had a few years back while trying to persuade a national newspaper syndicate to run a walking column. A skeptical editor remarked, "A column about walking? That's like writing a column about sitting! Everybody does it. So what?"

Today that editor is eating his words. His casual "so what?" has long since been buried under the weight of scientific information that continues to attest to the physical and mental benefits of walking. He was right in one regard, though—everybody is doing it. The Walkways Center in Washington, D.C., estimates there are now more than 55 million people—about one-quarter of the U.S. population—walking for exercise and fitness.

Just as impressive is the number of prestigious groups urging people to walk: the American Heart Association, American Lung Association, Arthritis Foundation, American Podiatric Medical Association and the President's Council on Physical Fitness and Sports, among others. Senior citizens' groups are staging walking events, such as the "Bay to Breakfast" walk in San Francisco aimed at people 55 years old and older. In Massachusetts, the governor helped put together project "Keep Moving," which is designed to get older residents up and walking.

"More and more groups are realizing just how beneficial and safe walking is," says Marsha Wallen of the Walkways Center. "In time, you'll see even more organizations and businesses encouraging people to walk and offering endorsements."

That isn't surprising when you consider how good walking is for the total body. From lungs to legs, from back to brain, walking is the best way to keep the entire body finely tuned and trim, as millions of health-conscious and weight-conscious folks are finding out.

"Brisk walking balances the major muscles and brings your body into better alignment," says E. C. Frederick, Ph.D., of the Pennsylvania State University Center for Locomotion Studies, who is coauthor of *Walk On: A Tool Kit for Building Your Own Walking Fitness Program.* "There's more upper body movement than there is in running. It's a unique exercise with its own special qualities that make it valuable."

Muscles in Motion

Consider all the good things that happen to so many below-the-belt muscles when you walk. When you take a good stride, your pelvis shifts, your buttocks muscles contract and the lead leg pulls you forward as your trailing leg pushes, a process that alternately flexes and relaxes front and back leg muscles.

As your hips stretch forward and backward with each stride, they also move from side to side so your trailing leg can swing by. This action works on your hip muscles, keeps your hip joints flexible and makes them tug rhythmically on your lower abdominal muscles, all of which could lead to a flatter tummy, Dr. Frederick says.

Muscles in your shins and toes lift your toes and flex your ankles so your heel can strike the ground.

Above the belt, as you pump your arms with each stride, you're building the flow and rhythm of walking. You're also constantly contracting and relaxing different sets of muscles in your shoulders and forearms with each movement. Plus, each time you swing a leg around in front of you, muscles in your abdomen, side, back and chest contract to hold your body erect.

On top of this, the more vigorous breathing expands your chest and lungs and activates your diaphragm, abdomen and ribs.

"Walking also affects the spine in positive ways," says Dr. Frederick. "It strengthens muscles in the pelvis and lower back, which may help some people with back problems."

Help indeed. An informal poll of 492 people with a variety of back problems showed that "walking was helpful in the long run for 98 percent of survey participants who make it a regular part of their routine." Many of those polled said they believe walking makes their backs stronger and more flexible and improves overall muscle tone.

Walking at least two miles a day was one of the 25 most-often-mentioned ways of easing back pain. The respondents also noted that walking at least 30 minutes a day four times a week greatly reduces stress, a major contributing factor to back pain.

While the survey didn't address weight loss, it's safe to assume that more than a few of the backache sufferers shed a pound or two while seeking pain relief, because walking is a great way to lose weight.

A 150-pound man, for instance, can burn 72 calories per mile while walking three miles an hour. Up the rate to four miles an hour, and that same man can burn 95 calories with each mile stepped off, according to Bryant Stamford, Ph.D., director of the Exercise Physiology Laboratory at the University of Louisville School of Medicine in Kentucky.

Add Weights and Burn More

If you want to burn even more calories and increase your level of aerobic fitness in the process, try hand weights. "Use hand weights during walking and you can burn more calories per mile than you would while running," says Dr. Stamford. Our 150-pound man, for example, could lose 126 calories a mile while walking three miles per hour or 134 calories a mile when walking four miles per hour if he carried 5-pound weights. If he drops the hand weights and runs at a pace of six miles per hour, he'll burn only 120 calories each mile.

If you opt for hand weights, Dr. Stamford suggests starting with two- or three-pound weights and gradually working up. Carry them with your arms bent and swinging. "Arm movements must be controlled because you can damage delicate elbow and shoulder tissues if the weights swing about indiscriminately," he says. Carrying weights at your sides or using a weight belt accomplishes little, because the weights aren't used actively in the walk. Ankle weights aren't recommended because they affect foot placement and walking style, which could lead to injuries.

Where you walk also affects the number of calories you lose. Walking in sand or freshly plowed earth can boost calorie burn by an average of 30 percent, according to Dr. Frederick.

You can also upgrade your calorie burn by walking uphill. At a pace of four miles per hour, if you walk up a 5 percent grade—a hill that'll rise about 5 feet for every 100 feet you cover—you'll burn about 45 percent more calories than while walking on a flat surface.

Naturally, the steeper the grade, the more calories you'll burn. But don't try walking up any pyramids at first. "Walking up grades is more strenuous than normal flatland walking and it strains your entire body, especially your cardiovascular system. A 5 or 10 percent grade should cause no problem, but a person should be in good shape to tackle anything steeper," says Dr. Frederick. (For perspective, consider that a 5 percent incline is about the steepest grade on a freeway, and stairs are about a 50 percent grade.)

When you're out walking your muscles into better shape and shedding those unwanted pounds, you'll also be doing nice things for the rest of your body. Take your heart, for instance. Walking gradually strengthens the heart muscle, so your heart pumps less and can rest more between beats. Walking helps cells use oxygen more efficiently, which is crucial for people with cardiovascular diseases whose impaired circulation may cut back oxygen supplies to the body.

Walking also seems to help prevent blood platelets from

clumping together and clogging arteries, a process that can lead to a stroke or heart attack. Researchers in Finland studying a group of men between the ages of 30 and 49 found that the blood of those who jogged slowly or walked briskly for 45 to 60 minutes five times a week had less tendency to clot. The scientists speculate that the mild-intensity exercise lowers levels of a blood component that causes clotting. Just as important, they note that these beneficial effects continued for a week after the men stopped exercising *(Circulation)*.

Walk Away from Heart Disease

The evidence continues to mount that walking raises levels of high-density lipoproteins (HDLs), the blood fats thought to protect against heart disease. Researchers at the University of Minnesota found that HDL levels rose significantly in obese young men who walked briskly for 90 minutes five days a week for 16 weeks.

"There's strong evidence that aerobic-type exercise, such as walking, does indeed raise HDL levels," says cardiologist James Rippe, M.D., director of the University of Massachusetts Exercise Physiology Laboratory and medical director of the Rockport Walking Institute.

Walking has a down side, but it's a good-for-you decline: It can reduce high blood pressure in some cases. Doctors at the University of Florida Hypertension Clinic in Gainesville have found that for some people, walking controls blood pressure better than drugs. They also report that patients with slight to moderate hypertension often see their blood pressure return to normal a few weeks after they start walking.

Bone density also improves as you walk, which is important to postmenopausal women who must be concerned about the bone-degenerating disease called osteoporosis. You may also find that your energy levels rise, because walking can increase the muscles' supply of glycogen (the fuel for physical activity).

Walking even works on your nerves, as evidenced when researchers at the University of Southern California, Los Angeles, asked for volunteers who considered themselves extremely nervous. Different means of relaxation were tried: a tranquilizer, a placebo (dummy pill), 15 minutes of walking at a heart rate of 100 beats per minute, and 15 minutes of walking at a heart rate of 120 beats per minute.

The test subjects found walking to be the best tranquilizer. Electrical activity in their muscles, which occurs with any normal activity but intensifies when tension rises, declined 20 to 25 percent after walking at both the lower and higher heart rates. The researchers concluded that walking is more effective and safer than tranquilizers, "and you don't have to worry about how it may interact with other medication you may be taking for medical problems," notes Herbert deVries, Ph.D., of the school's Physiology of Exercise Laboratory.

Creative potential can also be tapped through walking. "A brisk, sustained pace of about a mile every 15 minutes improves fitness levels, increases heart rate and gets more oxygen into the blood—all of which improve your clarity. And when there's less confusion and you can think more clearly, you tend to be more creative," says Joan Gondola, Ph.D., an exercise physiologist and psychologist at Baruch College in New York City. "We've found that as fitness levels increase, there are positive personality and mood changes.

"We're still not sure why all this happens, but the popular theory is that it's tied to increases in adrenaline or endorphins [chemical painkillers found in the brain]. We do know that the better your fitness levels, the greater your self-image and self-esteem. With women especially, we've found that as their fitness levels improve, they become more extroverted and have more friends. Of course, the fact that this kind of exercise helps clear up depression, anxiety and tension is also a factor."

What more could you ask from a total-body exercise?

Lose a Little More, a Little More, a Little More...

If Aladdin's lamp found its way into your hands, would you include weight loss on your list of three wishes? Do you feel nothing short of a miracle could make your unwanted pounds disappear?

The rub with losing weight is that we're usually better at wishing for slimness than attaining it. And sometimes we even try too hard, going on a rigid reducing regimen that eventually leaves our resolve limp as a rag. Here's another suggestion, with a lot less potential for backfiring: Take it easy.

"Your extra weight is the final result of many small behavioral acts, things like eating between meals or driving to places only two blocks away," explains Kelly Brownell, Ph.D., co-director of the Obesity Research Clinic at the University of Pennsylvania in Philadelphia. "So you can lose weight by making many small, clever changes—in diet, exercise and attitude."

For slow but sure weight loss, draft into your daily habits 10, 15 or more of the following little ways to lose weight. They're little because by themselves they probably won't make much difference. But together they can change your behavior just enough to get you eating better, moving more—losing more!

Go Grocery Shopping on a Full Stomach ● Nacho chips, doughnuts and other tempters won't have half the allure they would if you hunted through those aisles hungry.

Shop from a List of Necessities ● Allow yourself only one purchase that wasn't preplanned.

Take Only a Limited Amount of Money When You Shop ● As an extra reinforcement against buying high-calorie foods, limit the amount you can spend.

Invite Your Spouse or Housemate into the Kitchen ● When you're preparing meals and cleaning up, a friend on the scene will help to keep you from sampling as you go.

Don't Eat Foods Out of Their Original Containers ● You may think you're having "just a tad," but you'll probably consume more than if you had dished out the food in a measured portion. Better yet, don't bring your "weakness food" into the house in the first place. Present yourself with the hassle of going to the store for single servings if you can't fight off a craving. This way you'll either get some exercise (especially if you walk to the store), or you'll decide the snack isn't worth the bother after all.

Eat Only at Scheduled Times in Scheduled Places ● A regimen helps you avoid unstructured eating.

Use Good Plate Psychology ● Don't use place settings with intense colors such as violet, lime green, bright yellow or bright blue; they're thought to stimulate the appetite. The same goes for primitive-looking pewter and wooden plates. Instead, appease your appetite with elegant place settings in darker colors. Choose plates with broad decorative borders and a slightly "bowled" design. You can fit less food in them.

Have Someone Else Serve You ● Ask for smaller portions.

Police Your Eating Speed ● Put your fork down between bites. The slower you eat, the faster you'll feel full.

Establish a Time-Out Routine ● Halfway through your meals, take a break. One trick: Put a large pot of water on the stove when you sit down to eat. When it boils (in about 10 or 15 minutes), get up and make a pot of herbal tea. When you go back to the table, you probably won't feel like eating much more.

Chew Each Bite of Food at Least Ten Times ● This helps you really taste the food and makes you eat more slowly.

Don't Eat Everything on Your Plate ● Make it a habit to always leave a little food, unless you're having steamed vegetables and fish, or an equally good-for-you meal.

Leave the Table as Soon as You're Finished Eating ● Don't linger over the last bites.

Remove Food Stashed in Inappropriate Places ● Get the candy bars out of your desk drawer and remove the nut bowl from the coffee table.

Use Whipped or Softened Butter or Margarine ● You'll spread the flavor around using a lot less than if it was hard and you had to scrape it on.

Share Desserts ● If skipping them is unthinkable, split desserts with a friend.

Downscale Your Brand of Ice Cream ● If it'll be a cold day in Key West before your freezer doesn't have a carton of this confection waiting for you, buy the least expensive or a reduced-fat brand. Your intake of fat and calories will be considerably lower than if you ate the gourmet kind.

Don't Skip Meals ● You'll only overeat later.

Do More "Fidgeting" ● For those of us who habitually squirm, toe tap or finger drum, it has been found in one study that fidgeting burns up to 800 calories a day in some people. That's the equivalent of jogging several miles.

The problem, according to Eric Ravussin, Ph.D., visiting scientist with the National Institutes of Health and one of the study's researchers, is that "you really can't make your body have more spontaneous activity like fidgeting if you don't already do it. You can, however, decide to make your body work more whenever possible to burn extra calories."

"Try doing things like getting up to switch TV channels by hand instead of by remote control," he advises, "or putting frequently used books on higher shelves so you have to reach."

Swear Off Elevators and Escalators ● Take the stairs instead.

Fire the Maid ● Do your own housework. Depending on your body weight, studies show you can burn 195 to 305 calories for each hour you spend washing windows, mopping floors and doing other tasks.

De-automate Your Housework ● Make your body work harder. Wash dishes, mix batters and open cans by hand; hang your wash on the line instead of using a dryer.

Exercise during Television Commercials ● Those three-minute spurts will keep you out of the kitchen.

Go Dancing, Miniature Golfing, Bowling ● If you normally sit around and play bridge or watch television, do anything active instead. The most calories you can burn in an hour playing cards is 95, but waltzing can whisk away 195 to 305 for every hour on the floor, and an hour of square dancing can stomp away 330 to 510 calories.

Drink No-Calorie Sparkling Waters ● When you go out, find a substitute for alcoholic beverages.

Get Rid of Those Degrading Signs and Pictures on Your Refrigerator ● Don't use images of 300-pound women in bikinis or pink pigs on beach blankets to shame you into not eating. Your will power will be stronger from encouragement, not belittlement.

Hold a Conference ● Explain your weight-loss wish to family, friends or doughnut-bearing co-workers. Ask them to understand if you turn down their dinners or candy.

Learn That It's Okay to Say "No, Thank You" ● When other people offer you food, don't be afraid to refuse.

Set a Realistic Goal for Yourself ● "Take it one day at a time and don't punish yourself for slipping," says Suzann Johnson, nutritionist with Weight Watchers International, Inc. "You'll be more successful if you remember to be your own best friend."

How to Get the Most "Slimming Power" from the Rotation Diet

For those of you interested in losing 1 pound or 20, consider these words from a man who has a weight-loss plan to offer: "The first thing I want to say is, don't worry! You will be able to eat again like a normal human being and not gain weight! You will be able to return to the style of cooking you prefer (unless it's loaded with fat), you will be able to eat out, and while eating out, be able to eat as others eat."

So says the originator of the popular Rotation Diet, and they are delicious words to both the person considering his or her first diet and to the seasoned veteran of the dieting game who's tried them all to no avail. But in a nation where diets are consumed like salted peanuts, what separates this one from the rest that have come and gone as fast as a pizza delivery boy? More important, is it a safe, nutritionally sound regimen that works?

Experts say it's not an unhealthy diet, and you will lose weight, but only in the short term. The odds are that five years after starting the diet you'll have regained the weight you lost, possibly even a few pounds more than you had when you started, and you'll join the other 80 to 95 percent of the populace who fall off the diet wagon each year.

"This isn't an outrageously bad diet like some on the market, and there are no imbalances in the vitamins and other nutrients," says psychologist Morton Harmatz, Ph.D., University of Massachusetts, Amherst, who's spent 15 years studying weight-loss diets and eating disorders. "It's a lot like other diets that have come and gone, though, and all of them fail in several respects: They involve strict menus that no one can adhere to for long periods of time, which is what it takes to maintain weight loss. And diets like this don't address a person's desire for food or the root causes of overeating."

The Plan

The Rotation Diet is the creation of Martin Katahn, Ph.D., a Vanderbilt University psychologist who, after losing 75 pounds 22 years ago and keeping them off, decided his weight-loss plan might just be what a diet-hungry nation needed. (It's estimated that the average American attempts 2.2 diets a year, and on any given day more than 20 million people—mostly women—are trying to lose weight.)

For the first three days of the diet, you consume only 600 calories daily. Then the calorie count jumps to 900 for each of four days. In week two, you rotate to 1,200 calories daily for seven days. (For male dieters, add 300 to the last two figures.) The third week, you're back to 600 calories (1,200 for men) each of three days, followed by four days at 900 calories each (1,500 for men). If the 600- or 900-calorie rotations leave you famished, Dr. Katahn says, jump immediately to 900 or 1,200 calories.

After this 21-day cycle, you're allowed to stop and take what Dr. Katahn labels a vacation, which is partly designed to enhance your motivation. Chances are, he says, you'll prefer not to halt the diet. His reasoning is that you'll be so pleased with the rapid weight loss, you'll want to continue slimming down. Still, he stresses that the time out is crucial to success and insists on a week to a month off.

The vacation has limits: Don't exceed 1,200 calories a day for the first three days, or preferably a week, then move up to 1,500 calories each of three days, and then 1,800 calories daily for the remainder of your dieting hiatus. You can substitute any foods you want during this break—yes, even candy or ice cream—as long as you stay within the caloric bounds. You must drink eight eight-ounce glasses of water daily, which is also urged during the active dieting weeks. No low-calorie sodas, please, because he says they keep your taste for sweets alive.

Brisk exercise is mandatory. In Dr. Katahn's words, "If you don't get active and stay active, you've got a snowball's chance in hell of maintaining any weight loss." Dieters are to start gradually, about 15 minutes a day the first week, with brisk, vigorous exercise such as walking, swimming, gentle jogging, bicycling or bouncing on a trampoline. You should be up to at least 45 minutes a day by the end of the third week.

It's a mixed diet with a variety of foods, unlike the high-protein or low-carbohydrate diets that Dr. Katahn pans. Still, he advises that you may need vitamin and mineral supplements, and he stresses that anyone considering a fast weight-loss program should first consult a physician. The diet's not suitable for children and adolescents, pregnant women, nursing mothers and extremely active people, such as runners who jog miles a day.

Dr. Katahn says his diet increases your metabolic rate, which is the speed at which your body burns calories, and makes it easier to lose weight.

With most diets, the reduction in calories causes the metabolic rate to decrease. It then takes less food to create fat, and it's harder to lose the regained weight because your metabolic rate is slower than when you started dieting. (One reason for the vacation is that the slight increase in calories allowed during the break supposedly fuels the calorie-burning metabolic rate and therefore prevents it from slowing.)

Dr. Katahn allows little or no fat, sugar or salt, which may lend credence to some of the health benefit claims. He says to expect an average 10 percent reduction in serum cholesterol levels and a 15 percent drop in circulating triglycerides. People with high blood sugar are told they may see those levels normalize, and mild hypertensives might be able to reduce or eliminate blood pressure medication. The fiber in the diet's complex carbohydrates should "tangle up about 10 percent of the dietary fat you eat" so it will "pass right through your system without being digested."

You'll never get hungry on the Rotation Diet, says its originator, since you can stuff yourself with what he calls "free" vegetables—asparagus, celery, chicory, lettuce, parsley and watercress, to name a few of the 13 choices—that are low in calories but fiber and nutrient dense. There's also a list of all-you-can-eat "safe" fruits: apples, berries, grapefruit, melon, oranges, peaches, pineapple and tangerines. Pick only one type of fruit and stay with it, however, since eating several different kinds can stimulate your appetite, he warns.

On the average, expect to lose 5 pounds the first week, 2½ pounds the second week, and around 5 more pounds the third week, he says. The heavier you are, the more you lose, and if you're more than a few pounds overweight, Dr. Katahn suggests it's not unrealistic to drop 1 pound a day during the 21-day cycle.

Computer Takes a Byte

Which all sounds fine and good, but Kathy Musgrave was less than overwhelmed when she used a computer to compare 21 days of Rotation Diet menus with the Recommended Dietary Allowances (RDAs) for vitamins and minerals. "The diet is more than adequate for getting protein, but it's low in iron, zinc and vitamin D," says the registered dietitian, who is nutrition professor with the University of Maine-Orono School of Human Development.

The Rotation Diet supplies only 63 percent of the RDA for iron, 53 percent of the RDA for zinc and 31 percent of the RDA for vitamin D. "All the other nutrients are relatively all right," she says, "although they aren't up to 100 percent of the RDA. For example, the diet supplies 89.5 percent of the RDA for calcium for a 21-day cycle. Anything above 67 percent of the RDA is considered nutritionally safe. In any case, Dr. Katahn covers his bases by suggesting that dieters take supplements.

"Twenty-two percent of the calories in his diet come from fat, and the current national recommendation is that we get no more than 30 percent of our calories from fat, so that's a good point," she adds. "I'm concerned about the 600- and 900-calorie days, however. Even though it's only for a short while, it could be draining protein from the body's stores, so if your system is stressed or exposed to a virus, you may be more susceptible to illness.

"I'd recommend no less than 1,000 calories a day and more exercise. Instead of starting with 600 calories a day and 15 minutes of exercise, begin the diet with at least 1,000 calories daily and maybe 30 minutes of activity."

The Rotation Diet's emphasis on exercise is highly commendable, says Jennifer Anderson, a registered dietitian in the Food Science and Human Nutrition Department at Colorado State University, Fort Collins. But after studying this and other popular diets, she concludes that too little attention is paid to target heart rates.

"This is important for people in the over-50 age group, which is where a lot of dieters are, because they need special exercise programs," she says. "You don't have to get the heart beating to capacity to burn calories. You just have to speed up your metabolic rate by reaching your target heart rate." (The rate is computed by subtracting your age from 220. Sixty-five percent of the resulting figure is your target rate per minute, which you should maintain for at least 20 minutes.)

There seems to be some doubt as to whether the Rotation Diet actually increases the metabolic rate as Dr. Katahn claims. While some of the experts contacted felt the 600- and 900-calorie rotations would probably decrease metabolic rate, others said the calorie increases to 1,200 and 1,800 in the ensuing rotations may indeed prevent a slowdown. Plus, exercise is a scientifically proven means of stimulating the metabolic rate, and the Rotation Diet insists on brisk physical activity. As one expert says, "There's no data that I know of to support his claim, but there's none to discredit it, either."

As for the vacation, "it sounds like a psychological trick designed to prime you from the beginning, to give you hope that there's light at the end of the tunnel if you just hold on through those first three hungry weeks," says William Bennett, M.D., a Harvard Medical School researcher who's studied eating disorders and diets and who is coauthor of *The Dieter's Dilemma.* "I would guess the majority of the people will get off the diet at that point, however."

Says Dr. Harmatz, "If someone is overweight, you can't give them free rein over any type of food. People who overeat may do so in response to emotional needs, such as nervousness or depression. If you don't get to the root of the problem and solve it from that end, they'll just eat more and more of the so-called safe foods, until one day the safe foods don't satisfy anymore and they binge on high-calorie foods."

Needed: More Attention to Eating Behavior

Like so many other diets, the experts say the rotation plan is a Band-Aid treatment for a very complex problem. "These diets don't address the behavioral aspects of food consumption or the changes in lifestyle that are needed to achieve successful long-term weight control, instead of just temporary weight loss," Dr. Harmatz says. "Diets like the Rotation Diet give you a strict list of foods that are boring, especially when you think about them in terms of long periods. For any diet plan to work it has to be a commitment for extended periods. It's not a matter of losing 10 or 20 pounds and returning to old eating habits. If you do, the research shows you'll gain the weight right back—and maybe a few pounds more."

The diet made national news when cities, towns and neighborhoods from Colorado to Tennessee jumped on the rotation bandwagon and set mass weight-loss goals. Supermarket chains have also put foods for the Rotation Diet menus on sale and helped instill local weight-loss fervor. "The diet has gotten a lot of community support, and people get that initial boost of confidence and determination when they're in the grocery stores where the diets are being publicized," says psychologist Ron Powell, Ph.D., executive director of the American Institute for Preventive Medicine in Southfield, Michigan. "But when they get home, they're faced with the same old urges to eat, and there's nothing to change those behavior patterns that lead to overeating. Their confidence succumbs to temptation."

So is there such a thing as an ideal weight-loss plan?

"It's not a matter of opening a book," says Musgrave. "If someone is serious about losing weight, they should look at the diets available, modify them to suit individual lifestyles, and don't just accept them as is because that may not work."

According to Anderson, self-realization is the means to success. "Dieters need to discover for themselves what's causing their downfall. Do they eat because they're depressed, or are they habitual munchers who can't sit in front of the television without snacking? A lot of people don't think about how or why they gain weight. But once they're able to say, 'Oh yeah, that's why I'm eating so much,' we've found that they're more willing to modify their behavior and lifestyle so they can stick to a weight-loss plan. You have to take the responsibility, and not rely on a prepackaged diet in a book that worked for someone else."

Once you've found your culinary Achilles' heel, making changes in eating and cooking habits—baking instead of cooking with fat and taking smaller portions on your plate, for instance—is a major step. "Choose a variety of foods to make eating as interesting as possible, because boredom kills a lot of diets," says Musgrave.

"Drastic Changes Rarely Work"

"Drastic changes rarely work, so make them gradually," she adds. "Few people can go from a candy bar one day to a stalk of celery the next. It may take two to three weeks to get down to 1,200 calories a day, but that's all right because you'll be slowly making changes that can be easily integrated into your lifestyle with little stress."

Dr. Harmatz also favors a temperate approach. "It's best to cut back just enough so there's a calorie loss without disrupting the normal lifestyle all at once.

"Take people who want to lose 10 or 15 pounds, for example. They don't need a drastic plan, just a diet that's subtly deficient in calories. If you eliminate 100 calories a day, eat a few less slices of bread or one less handful of peanuts and exercise more, in a year's time you've lost about 10 pounds. The problem is that most people don't want to wait a year."

Exercise, as Dr. Katahn stresses throughout his book, is crucial to weight loss and control. Says Dr. Bennett, "Of the things that we can manipulate to make us lose weight, we tend to underestimate the impact of exercise. If people would just find some type of aerobic activity that they enjoy and do it each day for at least 25 minutes or so, they'll do more for themselves in the long term than any diet could ever hope to do."

Make Weight Loss Easier with Some Spouse Psychology

Susan looks in the mirror and groans, "I am definitely going on a diet."

"It never worked before, what makes you think it will work this time?" her husband, Bob, quickly retorts.

And then later that same evening, he eats ice cream directly in front of her, knowing full well that ice cream is the one thing she can never resist.

The next day he suggests they go out to dinner at her favorite, fattening restaurant.

"What's the use?" she says to herself. "I might as well not even try."

Yet there is hope. Susan may be able to get Bob to stop sabotaging her diet and actually help her lose weight.

Ultimately, the success of a diet doesn't depend on your spouse—it depends on you. But in some cases, having a supportive person around makes the difference between a diet that works and one that doesn't, says Kelly Brownell, Ph.D., associate professor in the Department of Psychiatry at the University of Pennsylvania School of Medicine and co-director of the Obesity Research Clinic, Philadelphia. Diet saboteurs may have several concerns, says Dr. Brownell, who is the author of *The LEARN Program for Weight Control*. "They may fear you will become too attractive to the opposite sex, you'll make more physical and emotional demands, you'll make new friends and have a social life that excludes them, or that you might become more competitive and independent," he says.

Getting the Right Kind of Support

Even when mates want to help, they may not know how, says Dr. Brownell. And so they take on the role of policeman, catching violations and doling out warnings. That can make matters worse. You get angry and tell your mate to mind his or her own business or you feel like a failure and eat even more.

The other person's negative comments may be his or her way of trying to help. But no one's forcing you to eat. You always have a choice.

You may find the strength to make the right choice despite those negative comments if you think more highly of yourself and put yourself first a little more, says Peter Miller, Ph.D., clinical psychologist and executive director of the Hilton Head Health Institute.

"You may need to take more time for activities that make you feel good. That could mean taking time away from other things, delegating responsibilities and getting some cooperation from your family," he says. And that's not always easy.

Your mate might agree, "You need to take more time for yourself, you need to exercise." But then as soon as you start to do it, he or she will say, "Just do this one thing for me first." So you have to stand your ground and take the time for yourself, says Dr. Miller.

If your mate seems threatened every time you decide to slim down, some reassurance may ease his or her mind, says Dr. Brownell. Sue could explain to Bob that she doesn't like the feeling that food controls her, she wants her clothes to fit better and she wants to feel more energetic. All the while, she needs to continue showing she loves him and keep from implying that he is responsible for her weight problem.

There are a number of other ways you can get your mate on your side, says Dr. Brownell. "The first is to communicate. Let him know that you'd like some help." Get a reading on your spouse's feelings about your weight problem and talk about how to best proceed.

Let your mate know what kind of help you need. Do you want to be praised when you do well or scolded when you do poorly? Should your mate avoid eating when you're around? Can he or she help by exercising with you?

Make specific suggestions about how your partner can help, leaving nothing to chance. Don't say, "Will you please help me?" Instead say, "It helps me a lot when you walk with me after dinner," or "I appreciate it when you don't eat ice cream in front of me at night."

Make the request positive. A negative request would be, "It makes it difficult for me to stick to my diet when you eat ice cream in front of me." A positive request would be, "Please help me by not eating ice cream in front of me." Positive statements make people feel good, and they respond better.

Finally, make sure you reward your partner for helping you. Don't expect the support and encouragement to flow only from your mate to you. Some of it has to flow back, says Dr. Brownell. Being supportive can be draining, so you need to acknowledge your partner's help. You've been receiving help, so do some nice things in return. There are many pleasurable rewards that you can give to your partner. Send flowers, buy your mate a new record, make Sunday breakfast, fix something that's broken, see the city or give your partner a massage.

If being direct and discussing how your partner's behavior makes you feel doesn't turn your mate from a saboteur into a supporter, then the best thing is to ignore it and get on with your diet, says Dr. Brownell.

When the other person heads for the ice cream, you may have to walk out the door and take a walk around the block. Or call a friend on the phone and start talking to get your mind off what's making you want to eat.

Giving Support

If you are in the role of supporter, how should you behave? Be upbeat and encouraging, says Dr. Brownell. You can say, "You look good, I'm proud of you," but don't push yourself on the other person. Ask your mate what type of encouragement he or she needs and how often. You may be surprised by what kind of help the dieter wants, says Dr. Brownell.

If your mate slips up a little and happens to eat something that's forbidden or doesn't exercise, don't respond with sarcasm or negative comments such as "There you go again," or, "You know you shouldn't be eating that." Learn to forgive and forget lapses.

You could be supportive by exercising with your mate. Take daily walks together. Or develop new interests that you can share.

Help out more. Make dinner or offer to get the kids ready for bed so your mate can go for a walk.

Be easy to please. Eat the same kind of foods so you don't have to fix two different kinds of dinners every night.

For more tips on successful dieting, alone or with a partner, you can order a copy of Dr. Brownell's book, *The LEARN Program for Weight Control,* by sending a check for $18 to Dr. Kelly Brownell, Department of Psychiatry, University of Pennsylvania, 133 South 36th Street, Philadelphia, PA 19104. Bulk rates are available.

Looking Good

The Best and Worst Tummy Flatteners

There's nothing more disheartening. You've sweated and sacrificed to take off those 20 pounds and now, after all that work, you ought to be svelte. But, apparently, nobody has told your tummy. Your belt still looks like the equator, and you're afraid your co-workers are going to give you a surprise baby shower.

The fact is, the sensible diet and the good cardiovascular workouts that helped you melt all that fat probably did little to tone your abdominal muscles, which are the natural girdle that keeps you firm in front. They often need individual attention—exercises that build up their strength. And they need that strength for more than your good looks. The four sets of muscles that make up the abdomen, working in concert with your back muscles, help you do everything from stand upright to sit tall. Anyone who has ever had a lower-back problem knows that the first order of business in getting the back in shape is to get the abs in shape.

But you also have to get your abs in shape without wreaking havoc on your back. Some abdominal strengthening exercises are anathema to those whose back muscles are also weak. While a fit individual can do straight-leg sit-ups until the cows come home, someone not so fit may find that pain equals no gain. You want to flatten your stomach, not wind up flat on your back.

For the best and worst of the common stomach flatteners, we went to the experts. In this case we asked the advice of Charles E. Kuntzleman, Ed.D., noted fitness author; Michael Yessis, Ph.D., an Olympic trainer who teaches biomechanics and the training of athletes at California State University, Fullerton; and Steve Smith, manager of corporate health and fitness at Coca-Cola Foods in Houston, Texas. Here's what they considered the best—and worst.

(And please note, beg our experts: These exercises will not help a protruding abdomen that's the result of one too many Pan Pizzas. Toning exercises don't whittle away fat—only diet and aerobic exercise do that. These exercises will, however, strengthen and tighten sagging muscles, which should make you *look* as slim as you can be.)

What to Do

1. The Abdominal Curl. Lying flat on the floor, keep your knees bent and your arms across your chest. Rise slowly, curling up each vertebra separately until you're at a 45-degree angle. This means your lower back should still be on the floor. Lower yourself slowly, which is a complementary exercise called the Curl Down.

The benefits: According to Dr. Kuntzleman, who calls this "the best exercise you can do," this simple movement uses only the abdominal muscles. Because you keep your lower back firmly on the floor at all times, you don't involve weak back muscles that could be injured. (Be careful, however, not to do this with your arms behind your neck. The temptation is to pull on your neck, which could damage those muscles, warns Dr. Kuntzleman.)

2. The Reverse Sit-Up. Lie flat on your back with your arms at your sides, palms down. Keep your knees bent and raise your legs and pelvis completely off the floor. In the final position, your knees will be almost above your face.

The benefits: This exercise complements the Abdominal Curl because it exercises the lower abdominals, says Dr. Yessis.

3. The Full Curl. Lie flat on your back with your feet close to your buttocks, your hands behind your head. Raise your head and shoulders and lift your knees at the same time, as if your head and knees were going to meet in the middle.

The benefits: Again, you are keeping your lower back on the ground, notes Smith, who teaches this exercise to his corporate clients.

4. The Pelvic Tilt. Lie flat on your back, or sit straight in a chair. Tilt your pelvis backward until your back presses against the floor or the back of the chair. Hold this position for 10 to 15 seconds, then release. Perform this exercise two or three times.

The benefits: It's an easy, simple exercise that anyone can do anywhere, says Smith.

5. The Reverse Trunk Twist. Lie flat on your back, with your knees bent. Lift your legs together at a 90-degree angle, keeping your arms out to your sides. Drop your legs first to one side, then to the other.

The benefits: You're exercising your internal and external obliques, V-shaped muscle groups in the front of your abdomen that are involved in spinal flexion and rotation, says Dr. Yessis.

6. Isometric Toner. You may do this standing, sitting or lying down. Simply pull your abdominal muscles inward and back toward your spine. Hold for a few seconds.

The benefits: You can do this anywhere, says Dr. Kuntzleman, and it's always safe and effective.

What Not to Do

1. The Straight-Leg Sit-Up. You probably did this one in gym class. You would lie on your back, with your feet flat and your hands behind your head, then raise yourself up to sitting position. Our experts also include Bent-Knee Full Sit-Ups in the no-no category.

The disadvantages: Unless you're in good shape, chances are you'll arch your back to get all the way up. That can hurt your lower back, says Dr. Kuntzleman. Besides that, he notes, you're using your stomach muscles only half of the way up, which is why the Abdominal Curl is the better exercise.

2. The Slant Board Sit-Up. If you use your local gym, you know all about the slant board. To do this full Sit-Up, you place your feet under the padded footholds and raise yourself up so you are doing a full Sit-Up in an inclined position.

The disadvantages: The same as Straight-Leg and Bent-Knee Sit-Ups. "I never recommend using this exercise," says Smith. "If it's done too aggressively, the hip flexor muscles are overemphasized. That can lead to pain problems."

3. Double Straight-Leg Raise. This one should also be familiar. Lying flat on your back, you lift both legs off the floor to various angles and hold.

The disadvantages: Besides putting pressure on your back, says Smith, most of the work is being done by your hip flexors, not your abdominals.

Relax Your Wrinkles Away!

Not all wrinkles are created equal. Some—like the sag lines caused when gravity pulls your brows or jowls down—can't really be prevented. But other wrinkles are not so inevitable. By changing a few bad habits, you may be able to forestall some major furrows.

"One of the most common types of wrinkles I see on patients are expression lines—such as frown lines between the brows—caused by continual overuse of the same facial muscles," says Jeffrey H. Binstock, M.D., assistant clinical professor of dermatologic surgery at the University of California, San Francisco. "Most people aren't aware when, or how much, they're using those facial muscles."

The constant use of other muscles in your body would tone the area, but not so on your face. "Expression lines deepen when you use facial muscles, because the muscles of your face attach to your skin, while every other place in the body, muscles attach to the bone," explains Dr. Binstock. "So, whenever you're frowning or smiling, you're also pulling at your skin. That pulls and bunches up the skin and eventually leads to furrows."

Everyday facial tension is a prime factor in the creation of expression lines. Most of us don't realize we frown or raise our brows when our face is tensed. So we rarely think to consciously relax our facial muscles. And it doesn't take a particularly stressful incident to make us tighten up those facial muscles in the first place. Simple eyestrain, talking, being outside with sunglasses that provide inadequate protection, or just concentrating can cause us to frown or squint without realizing it.

What can you do to prevent or help ease expression lines? "First, you have to learn to be conscious of the muscle tone in your face," emphasizes Dr. Binstock. "One way to do this is to keep a mirror by the telephone. While you're talking, watch the faces you make and you'll learn how these faces feel 'on the inside' when you make them.

"Relaxation exercises can help ease the strain on your facial muscles," adds Dr. Binstock. "Once you know how the muscles of your face feel when they're tensed, you can teach yourself to systematically relax them so that they feel heavy and warm. Concentrate on keeping your muscles relaxed for five minutes."

What about facial exercises? Because the muscles of your face attach to skin, most facial exercises are not worthwhile. According to Dr. Binstock, "What facial exercises do is basically re-create the same pulls that you're trying to undo."

A facial massage would be a better idea. "Massages are

HOW TO STOP WRINKLES IN A WINK

• Sleep on your back. Pillows or the mattress can cause creases on your face as well as a general tugging on your skin.

• Use a moisturizer. It won't remove wrinkles, but because dry skin looks more lined, a moisturizer can make lines appear less noticeable.

• Wear sunscreen daily. "I can't stress this enough," says Jeffrey H. Binstock, M.D., of the University of California, San Francisco. "If you go outdoors at all, wearing a sunscreen helps you avoid the leathery skin and crepey wrinkles caused by photoaging."

fine if they're gentle," says Dr. Binstock. "They feel good and can help you to relax, which is great. But massage won't undo lines that have already formed.

"What massage, like relaxation techniques, can help you do is to prevent lines if you don't already have them and perhaps ease some of the existing expression lines so they're less noticeable. Nothing short of cosmetic surgery can actually undo deep lines."

30 Tips
for Healthier Hands
and Nails

There's no magic to having beautiful hands and nails. Below are 30 tips that require only consistency and patience to keep your hands and nails fit and fabulous.

1. Use a mild, superfatted soap or a nonsoap cleansing bar for hand washing. Always rinse thoroughly.

2. Pat, don't rub, your hands dry.

3. Always follow with hand lotion. (If it feels too sticky for daytime, blot the insides of your hands with tissue and leave the cream on the outsides.)

4. When using lotion, always rub a little extra into the cuticle areas to keep them soft.

5. If your hands need extra moisture, dab them dry after a shower, apply moisturizer over damp skin, then wrap them with plastic wrap and leave it on for a full hour.

6. At night, apply a richer hand lotion or petroleum jelly to still-damp hands.

7. For an intensive softening treatment, wear cotton gloves over the moisturizer while you sleep.

8. Keep a small tube of your favorite hand cream in all the places you'll be reminded to use it.

9. To help keep cuticles shapely, gently push them back with a washcloth when you shower.

10. Don't cut your cuticles unless you have a hangnail.

11. If a hangnail does develop, soften it with cuticle cream, then cut it off with sharp scissors.

12. Use a sunscreen to prevent age spots. If you're using a bleaching cream, this is doubly important.

13. Don't undo all your good work. Wear lined rubber gloves whenever your hands are in water or exposed to chemicals (even household cleaners) or any other potential irritants. Always wear gloves outdoors in harsh weather—even on short errands.

14. Apply your favorite facial mask to your hands. Rinse thoroughly and apply hand cream.

15. A professional manicure once a month is one of the best incentives for keeping your hands well groomed. It also gives you an excellent start for a home program.

16. For strong, lovely nails, use your emery board to keep the sides straight (for extra support) and the tips slightly rounded.

17. Always file your nails when they're dry. Water softens them, leaving them prone to damage.

18. Use the fine side of your emery board or a diamond dust file for nail shaping.

19. Always file in one direction at a time, toward the center of the nail, holding the emery board at a 45-degree angle.

20. Keep polish on your nails to help strengthen them.

21. Always apply polish to dry, clean nails.

22. Use a base coat to add protection and help prevent discoloring from darker polish shades.

23. Don't remove polish more than once a week if you can avoid it. Learn to repair minor chips.

24. Touch up chipped nail color with two layers of the original shade. Then go over the entire nail with another coat of that color and finish with a clear top coat.

25. Use polish remover that doesn't contain acetone, which can be overly drying.

26. After removing polish, lightly scrub the nail and cuticle with a nail brush to remove the last traces of polish remover. Rinse and pat dry.

27. At night, soak nails in lukewarm water for five to ten minutes to help replenish lost moisture. Follow with a moisturizer rubbed into the nail and cuticle.

28. To bring up a natural shine, buff with a plain chamois buffer. There's no need to exert a lot of pressure. Limit buffing to once a month if your nails are thin.

29. Fingernails are not nature's screwdrivers. Don't use them to assemble bookcases, pull out staples or open packing cases.

30. Eat a nutritionally sound diet, which should supply your nails with everything they need to be healthy. While there are hereditary differences between people's nails—some are naturally thinner than others, for instance—if you have a serious concern about the condition of your nails, have your dermatologist check them.

Protect and Rejuvenate Your Skin

If you could buy a product that, with regular use, would slow down your skin's aging, ultimately keep you looking as much as 10 to 15 years younger and prevent skin cancer, would you use it? Well, that product already exists. It's called a sunscreen. And if you're not using one daily, you're setting your skin up for the premature wrinkles and sagging that are a result of photoaging.

"Photoaging," explains Gary Dugan, Ph.D., director of skin care research and development for Avon Products, "is the direct result of everyday damage caused when the sun's ultraviolet rays penetrate the skin and injure skin cells. The effect of this damage over a period of years is what many people think of as aged skin—blotchy, lined and leathery, with reduced elasticity. Brown spots that are mistakenly called age or liver spots are also aspects of photoaging."

"You don't have to be sunning for your skin to suffer the photoaging effects of the sun's ultraviolet rays," says Lorraine Kligman, Ph.D., assistant research professor, Department of

Dermatology at the University of Pennsylvania School of Medicine, Philadelphia. "Photoaging occurs even when you're walking around doing your normal activities.

"Part of the problem is that ultraviolet radiation is divided into two wavelengths that must concern us: UVA [the longer wavelengths] and UVB [the shorter ones]. It's true that UVA rays aren't as strong as UVB rays. [It's UVB, for instance, that produces a sunburn.] UVA radiation is present all day, however, from morning to sundown, instead of mainly from 10:00 to 2:00, as UVB is. So people who avoid the midday sun may still be absorbing huge amounts of UVA."

Although it's the combination of UVA and UVB radiation that is most damaging to your skin, UVA alone can, in time, cause your skin to age prematurely. Dr. Dugan emphasizes, "The message has to be that all sun exposure without sunscreen protection is damaging to your skin."

The sun's harmful ultraviolet light can even penetrate things you may have thought protected you, such as window glass and clothing made from thin fabrics.

"That's why, if you want to protect against wrinkles, you really have to use a sunscreen on a daily basis," adds Dr. Kligman.

Some Encouraging News

Not only can you prevent most photoaging, but your skin can repair some of the already existing sun damage. "Evidence suggests that if you start protecting your skin daily with a broad-spectrum sunscreen, skin that is already damaged will begin to repair itself," says Dr. Kligman. "If it is protected from further injury, skin builds a new network of collagen, its major structural protein, producing a new layer of connective tissue. Fine new elastic fibers form in this area.

"Much of this repair work won't be visible for a long time. What you will see, however, is that your skin's blotchiness may tend to fade.

"Unfortunately, your skin will never repair itself completely, but the best thing you can do to have a younger-looking skin in the future is to start using a sunscreen today."

How can you be sure you're getting the most out of your sunscreen?

"Be sure you choose a broad-spectrum sunscreen," says Lincoln Krochmal, M.D., director of clinical research for dermatology for Westwood Pharmaceuticals, Inc. "This means that it will block both UVA and UVB rays. It takes a separate ingredient to block UVA radiation. Look for the words benzophenone or oxybenzone on the label. This is the ingredient that blocks UVA. Remember that UVA rays are relatively intense even in the morning and evening, and only broad-spectrum products protect against them.

"Also, the longer your sunscreen lasts, the better. That means waterproof is an important quality. Here, the ingredients to look for on the label are polymers. They allow a product to stay on longer whether you're actually in the water or just sweating.

"If you have an allergy to PABA, which is the most common UVB blocker used in the formulation of sunscreens, there are perfectly good substitutes," adds Dr. Krochmal. "Try looking for a product that contains either cinnamates or octyl salicylate as the UVB blocker."

"I would highly recommend that people wear a sunscreen with an SPF [sun protection factor] number of 15 at all times," Dr. Kligman says. "For anyone with really sun-sensitive skin, such as redheads with extremely fair skin, I would recommend that they go for one of the newer products with an even higher SPF."

More Sun Safety Tips

Here are additional tips to help your sunscreen work more effectively.

● Find a sunscreen that you can also use as a moisturizer. That way it's easier to remember to apply it regularly.

● When you're going to be outdoors, in addition to your regular sunscreen, use a nonsensitizing, mild foundation makeup that contains sunscreen. Apply the sunscreen first, being sure you cover the places hardest hit by the sun, like your ears and nose. Wait until it's dry, then put on your foundation.

● Use a high-SPF sunscreen on your lips, because they do not have the same amount of natural protection as the rest of your face.

● If you've been out in the direct sun for a time, follow up with a mild, nonirritating moisturizer, especially on your face, arms and legs.

● Apply sunscreen to your hands and reapply it after washing them. You won't avoid age spots on your hands by using sunscreen on your face.

Remember, there's more to sunscreen benefits than protection against skin cancer—sunscreens are also the first line of defense in the fight against photoaged skin.

The Practical Psychology of Positive Living

Energize Your Memory!

The average human brain weighs about three pounds and is capable of retaining such diverse data as the multiplication tables that you memorized in the second grade, the details surrounding your first kiss and the price of a bucket of fried chicken from the local take-out.

So with such a marvelous memory tool resting between your ears, why is it so easy to forget about the gas cap and drive off from the pump-it-yourself station with it on the car trunk? Or forget an acquaintance's name, or misplace the car keys, or leave a package in a restaurant? Mere absentmindedness? Senility? Losing your mind, doomed to aimlessly wander the late-night streets, unable to remember name or address?

Hardly. Yet it's easy to fear the worst, especially when the years are sliding by. The comforting fact of the matter, though, is that memory doesn't have to fade at any age.

"A good memory isn't something fixed that you have or don't have," says psychologist Robin West, Ph.D., of the University of Florida in Gainesville, and author of *Memory Fitness over 40*. "Your memory for the past, as well as your memory for new information, depends on what you do to remember.

"The changes that occur as you age can be minimized. With training and practice, your memory can be substantially improved at any age. And you can take greater advantage of your potential ability, which is probably much higher than your actual level of performance."

The Name Eludes Me

Take names, for instance, which are probably the hardest-to-retain bits of data that we humans store in our gray matter. Names are difficult for several reasons. "When we meet someone, we usually hear the name just once," says Dr. West. "Also, most names don't have meaning in themselves. In other words, you don't have a way to associate them with common English words that you already know. My name, for example, consists of two common words and is easy to remember because you can say, 'The robin is flying west.' Anything that makes material meaningful makes it more memorable."

There are a variety of ways to sharpen your ability to recall names. The following are a few suggestions, one of which may work for you.

Pay Attention ● Often you're introduced to a person and discover minutes later that you can't remember the name. What may seem like a memory lapse is more than likely a problem with concentration. "To remember names, you must pay attention. This sounds simple, but most people rarely do it," says psychologist Robert Bjork, Ph.D., a memory specialist at the University of California at Los Angeles. "Introductions are usually made where there's a lot going on, such as at parties or meetings, and you're thinking about so many other things—how to respond to the new acquaintance, how to make small talk, or wondering if the kids are okay with the babysitter. Your mind's on everything except the name you just heard."

The solution: Listen carefully during the introduction. If the introducer speaks rapidly or mumbles, don't hesitate to ask that the name be repeated, pronounced slowly, spelled or whatever you need to have it clearly in mind.

"Learning the spelling of a name can aid your memory," adds Dr. Bjork. "Or asking questions helps. With a name like Bjork you could ask, 'Is that Scandinavian?' or 'Is that like Bjorn Borg?' It's an unfamiliar name, but linking it to familiar things already in your memory will help you recall the name later. And most people are flattered when you show that much interest in their name."

Repeat the Name ● Keep the name in front of you the entire time the new face is before you. Look at the person's face as he or she speaks and say the name to yourself over and over.

"Use the name out loud if you get a chance," Dr. West advises. "Look for an opportunity to introduce your new acquaintance to someone else, or ask a question, such as, 'What do you do for a living, Mr. Jones?' "

Use the Name ● How embarrassing to discover that you're unable to introduce someone you've known for years because you can't remember the friend's name. The reason may be that although you see the person often, you rarely use his or her name.

"Don't get into the habit of ignoring names," says Dr. Bjork. "When you see someone you know, say hello by name, or at least say the name to yourself to keep it alive in your memory."

Set Goals ● Large gatherings often pose a problem because you meet so many new people. Dr. West warns not to expect too much of yourself, though, and set goals of only about three to five names to retain. "Use your personal priorities to decide whom to remember. Pick those people you'll probably be seeing again, such as new neighbors."

Dr. Bjork says the act of recalling helps implant a name firmly in mind. "We've found that if you pause and recall a new name after about 15 seconds, then again in a few minutes, then in 45 minutes, and once again about three hours later, this retrieval process actually reinforces it in your memory. It even works when you're meeting a lot of new people, and it's not as difficult as it sounds. It just takes a little practice."

Use Mental Pictures ● Another hint—uncomplimentary as it sounds—is to repeat a new name to yourself while noting a prominent facial feature, such as a receding hairline, double chin or big nose, making sure this feature is embedded in your mind.

"Even if your imagery attempt isn't very successful, the

effort you make to form the image may help you remember the name and face," adds Dr. West.

Think of Name Sentences ● With the name sentence technique, the sentence elaborates or builds on a name to make it more meaningful. For instance: Alice Brady, she's always braiding, or George Beatty, what a gorgeous beauty, or Mr. Carrasquillo, drives a car that squeals. The name will come more readily to mind if the sentence is in the correct order.

"This method forces you to remember more words than just the name itself, but the additional words create a larger image that makes sense. If the sentence is meaningful as a unit, it easily brings the whole name to mind," Dr. West says.

"While some of these suggestions may seem absurd, making the name stand out makes it easier to remember," she adds. "Eventually you'll find that the whole process will come faster and easier."

And, for those fateful moments when nothing—not even prayers—will summon up a name from the far reaches of your memory? "Don't panic, because anxiety interferes tremendously with the memory process," Dr. West says. Take a deep breath, relax, and often the name will surface. If not, try to recall the situation where you two first met, or who introduced you, or what you talked about, because the associations may jog your memory.

"Nine out of ten times this works," she says. For that uncomfortable tenth time when all systems fail, however, "People aren't usually too upset if you forget a name, because they do it, too. Besides, if you forget it once and have to go through all of this trying to remember, chances are you'll never forget that name again."

Lost and Found

Consider what's probably an all-too-familiar scenario: You're almost out the back door when the front doorbell chimes. You're headed that way when the telephone rings, and in the mad dash to answer both you put your car keys down. When all is said and done, you aim for the back door again, only to discover you can't find the keys.

Such annoying episodes usually occur because we're doing one thing while thinking about something else. The solution is to train yourself to be conscious of your actions.

"Take an extra second to put the keys somewhere sensible, such as in the door lock so you'll see them when leaving," says Dr. West. "Or look at them as you set them down, and make a mental picture of where you put them. Be consciously aware of their location and tell yourself, 'I'm putting the keys on the mantel.' " The same holds true for gas caps placed on the car roof or on top of the pump at a service station.

Around the house or office, keeping things in their proper place reduces the demands on your memory. "Many people think they're scatterbrained or losing their memory because they can never find anything, when the real problem is that they're poorly organized," says Dr. Bjork.

One way to organize is to establish what Dr. West calls a memory place—a table by the door, your nightstand, or perhaps the desk; somewhere you'll place your everyday articles, such as glasses, wallet, keys or briefcase. You can also put reminder notes in your memory place to help remember tasks for the next day.

Away from home, consciously establish a memory space at a friend's house or in the hotel to avoid searching later or leaving something behind. In restaurants, where so many umbrellas, satchels and shopping bags are left behind, Dr. Bjork suggests, "If you're carrying an umbrella, that means it's probably raining and other people at the table also have umbrellas, so put them together in one spot. At least one person's bound to remember and remind the others.

"With a briefcase or bag, place it near the chair so it's almost in the way. Or lean it against the chair leg, so when you leave it falls and you notice it."

For those times when there's no practical memory place—at a party, for instance—place your belongings to the right or left of the first chair you see while walking into the room. When leaving, you'll notice that chair and remember to collect your items. To remember your coat, use mental imagery and imagine the entrance door wearing a large coat, so the image will come to mind as you leave.

But some people just don't like games and may feel frustrated and baffled by memory systems. "It's true in some cases," says Dr. West. "But if you just try to learn even part of a technique, you'll benefit and have a better memory. And if you practice, these systems stay with you.

"It'll take an older person longer to learn the procedures, and they are limited by this factor, but once they learn one of these systems, it will stay with them just as long as it will a younger person."

"All Pain and No Gain"—The Trap of Perfectionism

To the class, it seemed like a harmless question.

"What about the brain waves of dolphins?" came a student's query from the back of the room.

The teacher, in graduate school after raising three children, seemed shaken. She didn't know the answer. She stared at the floor and wondered, for the third time that week, why she ever thought she deserved to get a master's degree. She was too stupid. And now the whole class knew it.

Two depressing weeks later, with the help of her therapist, she learned one of the most important lessons of her life.

She, along with millions of other people, had a nemesis called perfectionism.

You probably know some perfectionists—those self-made superpeople who crusade through life with sky-high standards but who are usually grounded trying to meet them.

"Perfectionism is the world's greatest con game," says Philadelphia psychiatrist David Burns, M.D., in his book *Feeling Good: The New Mood Therapy*. "It's a concept that doesn't fit reality."

What it does fit is the distorted set of beliefs perfectionists have about themselves.

Somewhere along the line, perfectionist people picked up the message that "love, respect and reward will be theirs, if only they can be bigger and better and more wonderful than they actually are," Dr. Burns says.

A Breed Falling Apart

When perfectionists connect their self-worth with success, the result can be a loss of happiness and satisfaction with life.

"This is one of the most common themes we see in therapy," explains Dr. Burns, who is director of the Institute for Cognitive and Behavioral Therapies at Presbyterian University of Pennsylvania Medical Center. Like Dr. Burns's patient who expected her cerebrum to be brimming with handy little facts on the brain waves of dolphins and other scholarly matters, "these people just can't live up to the unrealistic expectations they have for themselves. And when they fall short, they somehow believe they're a total failure and deserve to suffer."

That suffering often shows up as depression and anxiety, marital and sexual problems and difficulty forming and maintaining relationships. The pressure of perfectionism may also predispose some people to problems such as alcoholism, the eating disorders anorexia nervosa and bulimia, and obessive-compulsive behaviors.

Superseekers can be caped in different kinds of perfectionism. "Most perfectionists aren't like Tony Randall's compulsive character, Felix Unger, on 'The Odd Couple,' " says Scott Pengelly, Ph.D., psychological consultant for Nike and Athletics West. While Felix declared war on all imperfection, whether it was in his slovenly roommate Oscar, his job performance or his underwear drawer, "most perfectionists are just trapped by the illusion that they can achieve perfection in certain areas if they push hard enough, usually areas they consider extremely important," he explains.

Dr. Burns points out three places where perfectionism can breed.

At Work ● Dr. Burns once lectured to a group of insurance agents on the pitfalls of perfectionist thinking. The salesmen nodded in agreement and applauded when he was finished. This was followed by a rousing address from the president:

"People, we were number two this year. That's not good enough. Being number one is the only thing that counts!"

"Pushing for perfectionism may not be the winning strategy you think it is," Dr. Burns says. "Each perfectionist thinks it can help make for a better performance, when actually it cripples the person with procrastination, emotional misery and insecurity."

In a study of over 700 men and women, Dr. Burns discovered that perfectionists experience distress and dissatisfaction with their careers and personal lives. And he found no evidence that they were doing any better or making any more money than their nonperfectionist peers.

"Despite what we've been taught," he says, "perfectionism appears to be all pain and no gain."

In Relationships ● Many perfectionists fear criticism and react defensively because they just can't stand the thought of being wrong. This can alienate others, resulting in conflicts in marriage and professional relationships.

In the Bedroom ● Although occasional impotence is normal, perfectionists may turn this into a catastrophe with the ego- and erection-deflating attitude, "Unless I'm a great lover, I'm less of a man." Perfectionist women may place the same burden on themselves, basing their self-esteem on the girth of their thighs.

Another type of perfectionist is one Dr. Pengelly calls a "hope I" perfectionist. He sees many of these people in both athletics and business. The tendency here is to get so wrapped up in thinking, "I hope I break this record," or "I hope I can save this project," that all the worry wins out and the goal is lost. "Perhaps no mistake is uglier than the brutal concept, 'I am how I perform,' " says Dr. Pengelly.

When all of society appears to back up their be-the-best attitude, it can be hard for perfectionists to realize that they're only hurting themselves.

"Our whole society puts a premium on perfection," says Jim Quitno, pastor of Grace Lutheran Church in Spirit Lake,

Iowa, who's seen a lot of perfectionism in his 15 years of counseling.

"In the workplace, we push our people to work as fast as they can, and when they are working at peak capacity, we may call in an efficiency expert to see how we can squeeze out even more productivity.

"We are a culture in which parents go to Little League games, sit on the bleachers and criticize their child for only making it to first base. If he had really tried, he could have made it to second. We're never satisfied."

A Quest for Love

While culture may serve as reinforcement for perfectionism, childhood may well be the root of the problem.

"Many of the people whom I have seen have the idea that somehow, if only they were perfect, their parents would love them," says Asher R. Pacht, Ph.D., clinical professor of psychology and psychiatry at the University of Wisconsin in Madison. The child of a parent who gives either inconsistent, conditional or absolutely no approval may try harder and harder to "win" the love that's not being given.

One 35-year-old career woman Pastor Quitno saw came from another kind of home that can breed perfectionism— the supersuccessful environment. Her father was a dynamo both in the community and in the state legislature. Her mother headed all the best organizations in town. Growing up in this home, she was often praised for her accomplishments. But she felt that she had to measure up to the level of her parents' success and their high expectations for her. The fact that she's simply not as talented as her mother nor as aggressive as her father set her up for some guilt-building failures.

Patricia DePol knows the pressure of living up to superparents. A recovered anorexic, she is now assistant director of the American Anorexia/Bulimia Association and a firm believer in making children comfortable with success and failure. "I was aware of subtle feedback growing up," she says. "There definitely was pressure to perform. What I know now, and what all parents should let their children know, is that love and assurance shouldn't be connected to being perfect."

Building Back Up

Perfectionists need to learn self-acceptance and let the air out of their overblown standards. The trick is to change the no-win mind-set and think in more constructive ways.

In this book, Dr. Burns explains some effective ways to overcome perfectionism through cognitive therapy, an innovative form of treatment based on the theory that, "You will feel the way you think."

"You can break out of perfectionism by learning to identify negative thoughts, recognizing the distortions in them from perfectionism, and learning to substitute more realistic and positive thoughts," he explains.

"When I was helping the teacher who felt like a failure for not knowing about the brain waves of dolphins, we looked at what negative thoughts crossed her mind right after that class. She was thinking, 'I should have known that. I must be a lousy teacher.' She saw that those negative thoughts were illogical for several reasons: She had never learned about dolphins, she knew deep down that no one can be expected to know everything, and she could have easily turned the challenge to her into a challenge for the class by saying, 'That's a great question. Let's all research this and find out the significance of it.' Eventually, she learned to think about herself in a more compassionate and realistic way, and her self-confidence improved."

Costs Outweigh the Benefits

Another method Dr. Burns recommends is to write out a "cost/benefit analysis." List all the advantages and disadvantages of thinking about something in a perfectionist way.

Take the compulsive car washer, for instance. Every neighborhood probably has one: A person who insists on washing his car every Saturday, even when it's not dirty. For this behavior's advantages, he might list that, "It feels good to have the spiffiest car in town." And that's probably about it.

His disadvantages might read, "I have no time for softball anymore. I spend a fortune on cleaning products, and I should own stock in Turtle Wax. I get really upset whenever it rains. I wish death to all birds." It won't take long to find out where all the tension's coming from. Once a person realizes that perfectionism isn't helping, it will be that much easier to give it up.

Dr. Burns suggests conducting a mini-experiment, where a person refuses to give in to a perfectionist habit for a certain amount of time. This can be upsetting at first, but riding it out until the worst of the anxiety is over will gradually help the person realize he can tolerate being imperfect.

One perfectionist felt intense guilt if all the windows in her house weren't washed every day. Using Dr. Burns's refusal method, she would pick a day and not go near the windows. Every hour and then every day that she got by without washing them would bring her closer to beating her habit, until she was comfortable with a more reasonable washing schedule.

Pastor Quitno offers a substitute motto for the many perfectionists whose fear of failure keeps them from trying anthing new: "If anything is worth doing, it is worth doing poorly."

"That motto certainly violates our cultural stress on excellence," Pastor Quitno admits, "but it can help a perfectionist. I'll say, 'Can you win an Olympic medal for swimming?' 'No.' 'Then does that mean you shouldn't swim?' 'No.' Gradually, a perfectionist can see that even in the areas where he set such rigid standards, there will always be room for improvement— and inadequacy, too."

"Learn to celebrate smaller goals," suggests Dr. Pengelly. "Jack Nicholson thinks a movie is good if it has two good scenes in it. I think a ten-cut record album is a good buy if it has two really nice songs on it. If you don't go looking for perfection in yourself, you'll probably surprise yourself and find satisfaction."

And remember, adds Dr. Pacht, "True perfection exists only in obituaries and eulogies."

Are You a Perfectionist?

Just because your house is messy or your checkbook won't balance doesn't mean you don't have a streak of perfectionism somewhere that could be holding you back. Experts point to four behavior patterns that may indicate a deep-down desire to perfect.

Procrastination ● You put off giving a dinner party until you have perfected a soufflé recipe, installed new carpeting and repaved the driveway for the big event.

"Finished Product" Thinking ● You overlook the satisfaction from doing something, like organizing a fund-raiser, and aren't happy until it's all over and the money's in the bank.

All-or-Nothing Thinking ● You slip up on your diet and eat a plate of pierogies; you feel that one indulgence means you're weak, your diet is a total failure, and you don't deserve to ever see your toes again.

Mental Filtering ● You dwell on the bad reviews of your latest book and discount the success of your previous two that got you an honorary degree from a university and a spot on Johnny Carson's "Tonight" show.

Give Your Soul a Vacation to Remember

By Mark Golin

Raise your hand if this sounds familiar. Last August I went on vacation to Florida. While I was there I pulled my arm out of whack from too much tennis, imitated a cooked lobster from too much sun and gained five pounds from too much food. I got home the night before work started and was greeted at the front door by a gathering of envelopes reminding me that VISA, American Express and Gulf all wanted to have a word with me. By the time I'd gotten unpacked, watered the plants and hit the Solarcaine I had come to a very important realization concerning vacations—I needed one!

In our consumer-oriented society, vacation has come to represent two different things. At one end of the spectrum vacation means relaxation, a time to kick back and let the good sun melt away the memory of office memos piled high like snowdrifts. At the other extreme, vacation is a time of heightened consumption, daring you to eat what you've never eaten before amidst a whirlwind of palm trees and Fun Worlds.

But the real question is, can a vacation mean something more than a year of recreation crammed into two weeks? Is it possible to bring home a lasting sense of well-being rather than settling for fading tan lines?

In search of the vacation that leaves you smiling nine months later, I spoke with Dr. Stephen Shapiro, psychotherapist, author and vacation consultant to National Car Rental. I asked him (admittedly with some desperate self-interest) why people come back from vacation needing a vacation.

"The first and most common reason is that too much activity is crammed into too short a time," he said. "Sometimes when people feel that they're missing out on fun and excitement in their daily lives, they try to make up for it on vacation with a schedule that leaves them physically fatigued by the end of a week.

"Another problem is timing. When the daily grind is starting to wear you down, that's the time to take a break. Many people put it off and leave for that much-needed vacation only after they've dug themselves deep into a hole of depression and fatigue. By the time they do pack their bags, they find that they can't leave their troubles at home and can't enjoy being anywhere else."

Already pleading guilty to both of the above, I wondered if there was anything else that could go wrong. "Believe it or not," answered Dr. Shapiro, "people oftentimes don't really do the things they would enjoy doing on their vacation. It's not easy to be good to yourself, and many times people aren't sure what it is that will make them happy. The problem is that when there's uncertainty, preconceived notions of leisure then enter and take over. You're not having real fun unless you're sitting under a palm tree on the beach sipping a piña colada just like the person in the magazine or on television. Deep down you might not like the beach at all, but you'll go there anyway since you're not sure of what you really like to do."

Don't Get into a Rut

"Along these same lines, you also see people get into vacation ruts where they keep taking the same vacation over and over even though what once was enjoyable no longer rests and regenerates them," Dr. Shapiro said. "The security of tradition combines with a fear of new places and the unknown to keep a person from finding a new vacation place or activity that he might truly enjoy."

I was beginning to think it was a miracle that anybody ever returns alive from a vacation. Was there a cure for these vacation crimes? "Of course," said Dr. Shapiro. "People in this country are very work oriented, but when it comes to leisure they find themselves a little out at sea since there are no hard-and-fast rules to follow. When someone comes to me for consultation, the first thing I'll ask them is to remember something they really enjoyed doing. Hiking might be one answer. When I ask them how long it's been since they took a hike, the answer is 15 years. 'Fifteen years,' I say. 'Why so long?' And then there are all sorts of reasons: They've gotten into a rut and can't break out, or hiking doesn't really seem like a proper vacation. I urge them to try it again after all those years, and the results are usually good."

While the rules are not concrete, Dr. Shapiro does have some vacation suggestions to keep all of us smiling. If you've hit the same old swimmin' hole one too many times, for instance, but can't quite seem to give it up for greener pastures (i.e., you're in a rut), try hunting out new possibilities on weekend sojourns. It's not as expensive as tampering with your two- or three-week vacation, and you just might find something that really leaves you glowing. If not, you haven't lost all that much.

When you do go on the big one, the long stretch in August, try to come up with a conservative base of things you like to do. To that base add two new things you're going to try this year. Out of two you might only like one, but if you make this an annual practice, you'll find your vacations will evolve naturally with your changing interests and personality.

"Spontaneity is a key word to remember," adds Dr. Shapiro. "We are conservative organisms trained to work within daily schedules, and oftentimes we bring that habit with us on our vacations. There's certainly nothing wrong with having an itinerary, but you've got to keep in mind that you are not a slave to it. Change things around on the spur of the moment if you feel like it. For example, you've planned a full day of beach lounging with a good book. You get all settled down on your blanket with a cold drink, but the sun is too hot and the book really isn't all that good. Leave. Go do something else. Some people are determined to weather it out because they planned for that day on the beach and they're going to relax if it kills them."

Another good vacation move is a one-day buffer before going back to work. According to Dr. Shapiro, "People tend to think that they can just shift gears instantly, which isn't the case at all. If you go back to work right at the end of your vacation, you may find your mind and body still in vacation mode. That can result in some disorientation and confusion, and could account for that low feeling you sometimes get your first day back on the job."

When all is said and done, a vacation is anything that vacates the daily routine and allows other, hidden parts of ourselves to come alive and regenerate. With this in mind, take stock of yourself. Which part of your personality hasn't been out for a walk lately, but instead has been lying low beneath the daily hustle of your normal routine? What would make that part of you smile? If you're not too sure of the answer, talk to your best friends and ask them if they've noticed something that really made you happy. With a little detective work on your part, you might find some new ideas to make your next vacation one to remember with a smile rather than with a groan and a sunburn.

Let's Not Fight about It, Honey!

The song of your marriage is stuck on an angry note; arguments play over and over. What happened, you both wonder, to the harmony?

Chronic arguing can creep into relationships and turn everything, from breakfast to sex, into grounds for a fight. But experts who study relationships say just wanting to get along may put arguing couples halfway there.

"Most chronic arguers don't like to fight all the time," says Sven Wahlroos, Ph.D., a Granada Hills, California, psychologist and author of *Excuses.* "They just find themselves sucked into arguments somehow, have had it up to here and want to do something about it."

One type of couple is an exception, however, and may not want to change. "Some couples are conflict habituated and, on a subconscious level, actually enjoy fighting," explains Suzanne Pope, Ph.D., clinical director of the Colorado Institute for Marriage and the Family. "Arguing is the style they prefer.

"Although they might complain bitterly, if you look at them they almost seem to be having fun. Conflict has an important function in their relationship—it's a way for them to get closer. Conflict, after all, does have a kind of passion to it when there's not intense anguish laced in," says Dr. Pope.

If, after some soul-searching, you decide you really do want to stop bickering, the next crucial step is to discover why there's friction.

Getting to the Bottom of It

Most barbs, insults and movable objects hurled in anger are launched for a reason. "There are lots of solvable problems that could be underlying chronic conflict between a couple," says Dr. Pope. Here are some to consider.

Poor Communication ● It causes wars, disasters and business foldings, and it is often at the root of constant arguing. "A good chunk of the problem is that these people don't know what's really going on with each other," explains Dr. Pope. "They have no idea of what makes their partner tick." One spouse may never have realized the other longed to have a child, for instance, and the subject was never discussed.

Boredom ● "These couples simply keep going round and round with fights because they don't know what else to do,"

Dr. Pope notes. "You've seen these couples out at dinner—it's just dead between them, and to avoid deadness and boredom they'll pick a fight because it's better than nothing; it is at least some kind of connection."

"Playing Old Mental Tapes" ● "Freud called this repetition compulsion," says Dr. Wahlroos. "The person subconsciously tries to work through some disturbing behavior or pattern he experienced in childhood." The unresolved conflict gets repeated over and over in the present relationship. A woman who was overprotected by her parents, for example, might create conflict in her adult relationships to avoid the risk of being too close, being smothered again.

"You continue to play out the same problem until there is some 'ah-HA!' experience through arguing that may tip you off to the real issue," adds Robert Kerns Jr., Ph.D., assistant clinical professor of psychology in psychiatry at Yale University School of Medicine, New Haven, Connecticut. "An objective third party, someone who's supportive of the relationship, might also be helpful to provide a clue to why you're really arguing so much."

Masking ● "When two people have a major issue unresolved between them, they'll mask it and fight about something they feel is more resolvable," explains Dr. Pope. The fight may be over something petty, like where to go for the weekend, but it doesn't cause as hopeless a feeling as fighting about something major, like a disastrous sex life.

Displaced Anger ● "This is triangulating," says Dr. Pope. "A gets upset with B but takes it out on C—C usually being the spouse."

Distance Regulation ● This can happen to couples who don't give each other enough room to breathe. One partner will create an argument with the subconscious hope that it will force the other to declare a short physical or mental retreat ("I'm sleeping on the couch!").

Boundaries ● Couples who allow too many people to crowd their lives may argue when they feel, "There's no time for us." "It's as if they're trying to be private in the bedroom with 20 people milling in and out," jokes Dr. Pope. Too private an existence, on the other hand, can make a couple feel as if they're stuck inside an egg. These couples consequently argue in an attempt to break the walls down.

Accumulated, Unresolved Resentment ● If a wife refuses to approve her husband quitting the corporate world to start an ice cream business, for instance, his resentment may take the form of battle armor.

Hierarchy ● A power struggle may be causing friction between two partners, each of whom wants to be the dominant force leading the relationship.

Payback Cycle ● "This is like collecting Green Stamp books," Dr. Pope notes. Something annoys one partner, but instead of settling it when it happens, the offense gets pasted away until later, when it's brought up in an argument.

If any one of these underlying conflicts seems like it could be causing the sour notes in your relationship, either some do-it-yourself tuning or professional counseling might help end needless arguing. But it's crucial to note, says Dr. Pope, that one kind of relationship conflict is a different beast altogether.

Abusive conflict is mentally wounding to one or both partners. "You can recognize abuse by the highly emotional, almost irrational personal attacks one partner will make, hoping to hurt the other. There's rage going on here, not just normal conflict, and it calls for in-depth counseling," says Dr. Pope.

Peace and Harmony

Once a couple waves the white flag, a truce can be maintained with the following techniques for countering boredom, unresolved problems and poor communication.

Beating Back Boredom ● When a twosome turns tiring, try "wild cards" to fling the element of surprise back into your relationship and bounce bickering out, suggests Dr. Pope. Make a list of wonderful things you can do to surprise and delight your partner and print the ideas on cards. Every so often, pick a card and plan your project. The surprises can be anything from making a room glow with candles to pulling out an old, favorite album and dancing in the dining room.

Another way to rekindle interest: Find a common dream you both have and work toward making it a reality. One couple Dr. Pope counseled dreamed of a long vacation together in Cape Cod and grew closer while planning it.

Working Out a Deeper Issue ● "It's difficult," says Dr. Kerns, "but if you get some truly optimal communication going, you'll gain ground. This is not a dinner discussion," he stresses. "Rehearse your thoughts ahead of time, then set aside time to really get into the issue. State your problem clearly and assertively but not aggressively. This topic is too important to risk leaving out crucial information."

When you're the listener, says Dr. Kerns, be an active listener. Take notes. Repeat what was said to be sure you got the right idea. "Compromise is likely to be needed," he adds, "and it's an excellent skill to learn. Your goal is to end up on middle ground where you both feel comfortable, with parts of each of your needs met. This is tricky—lots of people hold stubbornly to the belief that only their own desires are valid. This gets in the way of really learning how your partner feels.

"You must remember that your spouse has needs, too. This is the bottom line of the last step—brainstorming. Come up with as many suggestions for solutions as possible. Somewhere on your list might be a good deal for each of you," Dr. Kerns notes.

Dr. Pope recommends a hard look at yourself if you're burning to change some behavior of your partner's. "You shouldn't be so dependent on this change that you think, 'Oh, if this doesn't stop, my life is going to be destroyed,'" she says. Try removing yourself from whatever it is about your partner that heats up your blood.

"When you push people into being any certain way, they'll dig in their heels and resist you like crazy. While you can express your desire for things to be a certain way, you need to be willing to let go and surrender to the fact that they may stay the way they are."

Dr. Wahlroos points to trust—or lack of trust—as being at the center of many couples' arguing. "Whether it's who will pay the bills, who will decide how to discipline the kids or how the in-laws will be handled, it comes down to partners not trusting the other's judgment," he says.

"Couples never think about this because they get so locked into the actual content of the disagreement and don't see what's behind it. In therapy, or together at home, that mistrust has to be challenged.

"An effective challenge," Dr. Wahlroos says, "is to think, 'Suppose I die today? Would my spouse be able to raise the children well, or would they end up delinquent? Would he or she handle the finances, or would everyone end up in the poorhouse?'

"That thinking will usually bring an admission, 'Yes, he would manage,' or 'She's quite capable.' This then gives you something positive to work with—you know you have a solid amount of trust available."

Communicating to Defuse Disputes ● Learn more conflict resolution skills. Read books, go to seminars. "They really work," says Dr. Pope. (For more information, write to the Colorado Institute for Marriage and the Family, 528 West Pearl, Boulder, CO 80302.)

Take criticism constructively when it's dished out. By refusing to accept any blame or admit any faults, says Dr. Wahlroos, you encourage more arguing. The key: Don't defend yourself when accused. Put the burden of proof on the other person. If he or she can't support the criticism, exaggerations and unfair barbs get shot down. If the accuser hasn't been blue in the face for nothing—he can support his claim as well as Perry Mason—then you've learned something and can work on improving yourself.

Take time-outs. Set a 30-minute time limit to discuss things and then stop. Walk, garden or work.

Try forgiveness, and let go of resentment.

Make up for slip-ups. When you both agree to do something or behave a certain way, set up "payment," like giving a back rub or cooking dinner that night for the injured spouse when one of you falters.

Finally, keep a sense of humor. See how self-destructive it is to squabble so much. After all, you wouldn't argue all the time with a good friend. And your partner is, first and foremost, a good friend.

A Jug of Wine, a Loaf of Bread, and You Can Forget All about *Thou*

Tom and Brenda planned a big evening on the town to celebrate their first anniversary. They had dinner at their favorite French restaurant, where the bordelaise sauce flowed like wine, specifically like the two bottles of Dom Perignon champagne Tom extravagantly bought for the occasion. After dinner, they held hands in the candlelight, sipping brandy and picking at the luscious French pastries the waiter brought around on the cart. It was the most romantic evening either of them had spent and they were both anxious to get home to make love. But once they were in bed, Tom found that not only couldn't he get an erection, once his head hit the pillow he had forgotten why he wanted to.

•   •   •

Bill and Helen have been married for about 15 years. In the early part of their relationship, their sex life had been something to write home about. But lately, it's been strictly something for the dead letter office—as is the rest of their marital relationship. Since Helen started working as a part-time office clerk to bring in extra money, they've been at each other like a remake of "The Bickersons." Lately, Bill hasn't been much in the mood for love.

•   •   •

Those two scenarios illustrate that, as psychologist and sex expert Albert Ellis, Ph.D., says, male sexuality is "a sensitive thing," subject to the vagaries of a man's lifestyle, his relationships and the occasional overdone dinner date.

Of course, having a breakdown in the bedroom once in a while is not abnormal. In fact, says noted sex authority William Masters, M.D., it's the rule rather than the exception. The enemies of male sexuality are legion. "It's the rare man who reaches the age of 50 and functions perfectly on every occasion . . . and the rare woman, too," says the physician who, with his wife, Virginia Johnson, pioneered modern American sexual research and founded the famous Masters and Johnson Institute in St. Louis.

Physical and Mental Factors

The two major failures of male sexuality are impotence (inability to get or maintain an erection) and loss of libido (sexual desire). For many men who experience one or the other or both, the causes are physical. Diseases such as diabetes and atherosclerosis may seriously undermine a man's love life. So can many blood pressure drugs and even antihistamines.

As Tom discovered, too much alcohol and even overeating can also ruin your best sexual plans for the evening. But perhaps the fiercest enemies of male sexuality lurk in what Dr. Masters calls the "primary erogenous zone," the brain.

Job stress, anger, discord in a relationship, depression, fears of intimacy, even worry can interfere with a fulfilling love life. In fact, any blow to a man's self-esteem can act as effectively as a cold shower. And often, it's that one amorous failure—for whatever reason—that does in a man's sexuality if he believes it gives him even the merest cause for self-doubt.

Says Dr. Masters, "It's fair to say that any man who has one single occasion to seriously question his sexual capacity is well on his way to impotence. Notice I don't say one single occasion of not functioning, but one single occasion of *seriously* questioning his ability to function."

He provides an example. "We had a set of identical twins who celebrated their fortieth birthday together. They went out and both men had too much to drink, so their wives had to drive them home. Both men tried to have intercourse that night and they both failed. The next day one apologized to his wife and said, 'Gee, I'm sorry dear, I had too much to drink. I'll make it up to you.' The other said, 'Gee, I wonder what's wrong with me?' and he became impotent."

The first twin realized that, of course, it was his drinking that wilted him sexually. Scientific studies show that alcohol, to borrow from Shakespeare, provokes desire but takes away performance. The second twin? He became a victim of that self-fulfilling prophecy known as performance anxiety: "I'm afraid I can't, therefore I can't." Men who fall victim to performance anxiety not only experience psychological impotence but in many cases lose their desire for sex, an unfortunate double whammy.

"If a man is worried that he can't perform, his drive will diminish. It's a defensive process," explains Peter A. Wish, Ph.D., director of the New England Institute of Family Relations, Framingham and Brookline, Massachusetts. "If he doesn't feel like having sex, he doesn't get into a situation where he can fail."

Perhaps the greatest enemy of a man's sexuality is our culture, the one that spawned the sexual revolution and now grapples with herpes. Many men are handicapped by a collection of unquestioned cultural myths. Dr. Masters calls them the "thou shoulds."

"Many women are well aware of the inhibitions they had as young girls from the 'thou should nots,' " says Dr. Masters. "But what most of us aren't aware of is that the male experiences something similiar that may bring him greater trauma. A man is handicapped by the 'thou shoulds.' "

They are, in brief, thoroughly intimidating expectations that no man can live up to. The man who tries may find that he falls short in more ways than one.

"For instance," says Dr. Masters, "the man is supposed to be the sex expert. Well, you know he isn't. The only man I know who is an expert on female sexuality is the man who knows he doesn't know. He's supposed to have infinitely greater demand, drive and capacity than a woman. Nothing is further from the truth. Human females have infinitely greater physical capacity to respond sexually than the man ever dreamed of. It's comparing apples and oranges. And when he tries to put as many marks on the wall as a responsive partner, he's in trouble. Finally, he thinks he's supposed to 'do' for the female. If she's not orgasmic, it's his fault. That's a complete denial of sex as a natural function. No man can make a woman be orgasmic. He can aid and abet, but he can't do for her any more than she can ejaculate for him."

Great Expectations

Other myths fall into the "great expectations" category. "Some people have unreal expectations regarding sex," says Jack Jaffe, M.D., director of the Potency Recovery Center in Los Angeles. "The best example is the couple who causes loss of libido by waiting for 'the great moment.' They're just not going to have it until everything is perfect. Well, they can be waiting ten years for that 'great moment.' They never really give it a chance to get started. That's one way they turn off their libido."

Another "great expectation" of both men and women is that a man should be "on" all the time, no matter if he has worked 22 hours that day, run a marathon or lost his best friend in a traffic accident—three nearly surefire ways, the experts say, to bring on temporary sexual difficulties. "Too many men uncritically accept these superhuman standards and then get concerned when they discover they're human," says Dr. Wish. "Men have to perform. Or, at least, that's their perception of it. When they get into a situation where all systems aren't go, they have a problem."

Men, says Dr. Jaffe, have to realize they have an "off" button, too, and it's just as natural as the one marked "on." "A man can't keep thinking that he has to put in a hard day at work and come home and perform sexually. That's not the way it works in real life. Now, the guy who's 25 may be able to do it. The guy who's 35, maybe he can, too. But as he passes 45 and heads toward 55, he's going to be in big trouble if he doesn't change those mind-sets of what he's 'supposed' to be."

Age brings with it certain physiological changes that may alter both a man's sexual appetite and his abilities. A man may find problems either if he doesn't acknowledge those changes as natural, or if he believes, as many men do, that advancing age is the slowly lowering curtain on his sex life.

"A 65-year-old man decides to have a footrace around the block with his 16-year-old grandson. If he beats the grandson, he worries about the grandson, doesn't he?" says Dr. Masters. "But if he doesn't have an erection as fast at 65 as he did at 16, he says, 'What's wrong with me?' He never thinks that every other natural function slows in its efficiency by the time the male reaches his late fifties or early sixties. He just thinks sex is different. And if that's what he thinks, he's handicapped."

He's just as handicapped if he thinks, as many men do, that sex is an activity reserved for the young. Nothing could be further from the truth. Although there are changes, says Dr. Masters, "The only things a male needs for effective sexual function in the 80- to 90-year age group is, one, a reasonable state of general good health and, two, an interested and interesting partner. And that's all."

Intimate Strangers

Douglas H. Sprenkle, Ph.D., director of the Purdue University Marriage and Family Therapy Program, has identified three types of couples conflict that frequently lead to loss of libido. They are the need for balance between closeness and distance, power struggles and territorial disputes. Ironically, says Dr. Sprenkle, all three actually serve a purpose in a relationship.

"Taking control, for example. If someone feels powerless in a relationship, one possible way to regulate control would be by not being interested in sex," he points out. "One of the goals of therapy is to help couples find ways of regulating these things other than through inhibited sexual desire."

The closeness/distance issues are some of the more frequent desire killers, largely because people tend to have different intimacy needs. "An awful lot of men feel smothered by women with whom they're involved in relationships," says Dr. Sprenkle. "I've worked with a number of men who were hooked up with women who wanted to be with them all the time and insisted on more intimacy than they felt comfortable with.

"We worked with one college professor who lost his sexual desire during the week but not on the weekends. As it turned out, he wanted to be left alone during the week to do his writing and class preparation. This loss of libido often serves as a distance-regulating function."

The professor learned to handle his problem more appropriately by developing new, more acceptable ways of saying "not tonight, dear" that didn't offend or hurt his partner.

Anger and hostility are effective sexual dampers. A man who, like Bill in the second example above, is angry that his wife has taken a job without his approval—and who may even see it as a threat to his masculinity—may be surprised to find that not only can't he make love to his wife, he doesn't want to. Anger and sexual desire tend to be mutually exclusive.

"I would say that many sexual-drive problems are really intimacy dysfunctions," says Dr. Wish. "There might be anger, unresolved conflicts, any one of a number of things that are unresolved and incomplete. If they're deep-seated, the couple may need special counseling."

Sexuality's Best Friends

It's a wonder, given the hostile territory, that a man's sexuality survives at all. It does because, despite all these enemies, it has more than a few friends. One, of course, is the sex therapist, who may be a medical doctor, psychiatrist, psychologist or even a trained clergyman, who can help when the problems become too large and complicated for a man to handle on his own.

But there are plenty of things a man can do even earlier to keep this important facet of his life *alive.* Here are some of his best friends.

Feeling Good ● "Feeling good about yourself is the important thing," says Dr. Wish. Many sexual disorders are brought on by assaults on your self-esteem. If you care about yourself, think you're okay and have a good, open, loving relationship, you're well on your way to a happy, healthy sex life.

Making Time ● "One thing sex therapists teach is time management," says Dr. Jaffe. "Plan time for sex even if you're not really in the mood. You must learn to have boring sex to have good sex. Sometimes you have to do it and not have all the bells and whistles going off."

Dr. Wish recommends making dates for sex with your mate, which not only gives you the opportunity for a few hours of uninterrupted lovemaking but days of wonderful anticipation.

Worried about the kids? Says Dr. Wish, "You've got a bedroom. It has a door. The door has a lock. Kids aren't stupid. They may know what's going on. But maybe it's the best example you can give to show them that a husband and wife can be loving."

Touching ● "Somebody said you should have a good 20-second kiss three times a day to keep the relationship going," says Dr. Jaffe. "Little things like that will eventually lead to increased libido because you'll have the supportive effort of both mates. Try for a certain amount of hugging and kissing, and later on that's going to help build up the interest." The fact is, says Dr. Jaffe, sex comes under the use-it-or-lose-it rule. "You can lose the habit if you don't do it frequently enough," he says.

Talking ● "I'm amazed at the people who come in here who've been married 20 years and have never really told the other person what feels good," says Dr. Wish. Talking frankly with your partner can not only keep your interest up and promote closeness—by sharing you can improve the quality of your sex life. And sex, says Dr. Masters, "is one of the better if not the best means of nonverbal communication in a committed relationship."

Varying the Theme ● For some men, the greatest threat to a fulfilling love life is the rut they're in. "Change positions. Add variety and spice," says Dr. Wish. "Go away for a weekend. Ship the kids off to a friend's house. Move the bedroom furniture around." Do anything that will help you and your mate break old habits.

Having Fun ● "Sex isn't supposed to be work," says Dr. Wish. "It's supposed to be pleasurable. So have fun!"

Good Health: Take It—But Take It Easy!

After a few workouts that left you feeling ecstatic, have you ever plunged enthusiastically into a seven-day-a-week, bop-till-you-drop exercise schedule?

Has losing a few pounds made you feel so great you decided to keep going until you ironed out every last ripple on your body?

If so, you are not alone, but you may be asking for trouble. Anytime you go to an extreme on anything it's potentially harmful.

Don't be discouraged from pursuing a healthy habit, just be aware that we are all capable of overdoing anything that makes us feel good.

Here's where you may have stepped out of the bounds of moderation in your healthy habits and into overkill.

Exercise

"When you start exercising, you notice that you feel good," says Gabe Mirkin, M.D., author of several fitness books, including *Dr. Gabe Mirkin's Fitness Clinic*. "The tragedy is that the mood uplift you get from exercise lasts only from 6 to 18 hours. So you have to go back the next day and get your fix. Unfortunately, as you get into better and better shape, you need greater amounts of work to get the same uplift."

This has been called a positive addiction, but for some people, it's negative. "Many people become attached to the mood uplift and feel absolutely despondent when they miss a workout," he says.

Unfortunately for them, people who exercise more than

four times a week have a high incidence of injuries. The number of injuries in people who exercise three times a week or less is extremely low.

Every time you exercise, your muscles are injured slightly. But in 48 hours they repair themselves and become stronger. If you try to exercise before your muscles have recovered from their previous workout, you can injure them badly.

When you overexercise, you may also find you get frequent colds, develop an "I don't care" attitude, have frequent headaches, constipation, diarrhea or muscle and joint pain and swelling; women may stop menstruating.

If you want to keep exercising for the rest of your life, you should listen to your body's signals that you may be doing too much. And you have to set reasonable limits, says aerobics expert Kenneth H. Cooper, M.D., of Dallas. He suggests that the optimum amount is 30 to 40 minutes three times a week. A half hour five times a week should be the maximum for most of us.

If you do exercise two days in a row, play it safe by alternating activities. For example, walk, run or do aerobic dance one day. These use primarily your lower leg muscles. The next day you might bicycle, which uses your upper legs, or swim, which works mostly the arm muscles. Recent studies have shown the incidence of injuries is much lower in triathletes when compared to marathon runners who do just one sport, says Dr. Mirkin.

Obligatory runners (those people who "must" run) often restrict other pleasures they used to enjoy, says Alayne Yates, M.D., psychiatric professor at the University of Arizona Health Sciences Center in Tucson. Dr. Yates is just finishing a study on the similarities between obligatory runners and people with anorexia nervosa. Both groups are similar in their extraordinarily high self-expectations, tolerance of physical discomfort and denial of potentially serious injury. If you are one of those who has become obsessed with exercise, step back and take a look to see whether this is what you really want, she says. It may give you a sense of identity, a sense of being something and going someplace, but you don't need to be so constrictive. You need to "find yourself" in a number of different areas.

Dieting

There is no indicated medical benefit from weight loss for people who are already within the normal range, says Arnold E. Andersen, M.D., a psychiatrist at Johns Hopkins University School of Medicine, Baltimore, and author of a medical text on the treatment of anorexia nervosa.

Most of us diet because we want to look fitter, healthier or more beautiful. But even moderate weight loss can be hazardous to your health, he says. The 10 to 15 pounds you lose and gain repeatedly hundreds of times in your lifetime can make future weight loss harder and may predispose you to increased heart disease and other problems.

Losing a lot of weight in a short time can have a dangerous effect on virtually every organ in your body. You may also become apathetic and less sociable. And methods you might choose for losing weight, such as crash dieting, eating limited kinds of food, vomiting or using diuretics or laxatives, have their particular dangers, says Dr. Andersen.

If you really need to lose weight, be thoughtful about it, Dr. Andersen advises. "Decide on a reasonable goal and choose a method that's not injurious. People who try to do it quickly don't maintain it. The only thing that seems to work is permanent long-term alterations in behavior and eating habits—a combination of moderate calorie restriction, avoiding foods high in fat and sugar, moderate regular exercise and dealing directly rather than indirectly with stress."

Sleep

The popular notion that sleep is always good for us deserves a splash of cold water, says George Globus, M.D., of the University of California at Irvine. You may have heard that, if you want to be healthy, you have to get eight hours of sleep a night. But many people get by very well on much less snoozing.

"Often we think we need more sleep than we do," says Peter Hauri, Ph.D., director of the Sleep Disorders Clinic at Dartmouth Medical Center, Davenport, Iowa. "When you sleep too long for a day or two, you may develop insomnia because you begin to sleep less to equal out the excess. This disrupts your normal sleep pattern, which can lead to further insomnia.

"You can find out how much sleep you really need by reducing the amount you sleep each night by one hour for a week," Dr. Hauri says. "At the end of the week, ask yourself if you feel better during the day or worse. If you feel worse, try sleeping more. Alter the time up and down until you find out at what point you feel good."

"It's a well-established fact that one has sleep blahs with excessive amounts of sleep," adds Wilse B. Webb, Ph.D., of the Department of Psychology at the University of Florida in Gainesville. "Whenever you build up a need for sleep and sleep longer than your normal amount, you tend to be groggy and have a difficult time facing the world. A little less sleep is a lot better than a little more sleep in terms of feeling well."

Stretching

Do you dutifully stretch before exercising to prevent injuries? And when you're in a hurry, do you try to do it all in less time? Some experts now say you can forget the stretching, at least before you exercise. And if you're going to stretch in a hurry, it's probably better not to stretch at all.

Joseph D'Amico, D.P.M., New York City podiatrist and professor of orthopedics at the New York College of Podiatric Medicine, conducted a survey of 540 runners and found that the number of injuries in the lower extremities increased as the time of stretching increased. He concluded that, (a) people are overstretching, (b) not everyone who is stretching should be and (c) the warm-up is not as important as the warm-down.

Who should stretch? "People who are tight. People who are already loose don't need it," says Dr. D'Amico. "They need strengthening and tightening. Most of the time, however, those who are real tight don't like to stretch, so they don't. The people who can stretch, do."

Most people who get injured overstretch before their muscles are warmed up. If you do that, you could tear a muscle instead of gently stretching it. So the key to preventing injuries is always stretch after you warm up, says Dr. Mirkin. "The resting muscle temperature is 98°F, but with just a slight jog your muscle temperature will go to 102°F. Muscles are like furnaces. They produce heat and this makes them more pliable, like putty, and then you can stretch out."

When you do stretch, do it slowly and deliberately and stretch no further than you can hold for five seconds. If it starts to become painful, stop and let up. And don't bounce. Bouncing actually makes your muscles contract more to protect themselves and they tear more easily.

There is no evidence that stretching will prevent injuries. But there is evidence that it can help athletes who must do fast, explosive movements, says Dr. Mirkin. "Longer muscles will allow you to exert a greater force about a joint, which will give you greater power, which in turn will help you run faster, jump farther or higher. So competitive athletes should stretch seven days a week, but noncompetitive athletes should stretch only if they want to."

You certainly don't need to stretch to be fit, says Richard Dominguez, M.D., co-director of SportsMed Clinic in Carol Stream, Illinois. Jogging, walking, bicycling or swimming can all be done very safely without stretching. After a workout, however, stretching helps reduce soreness.

Once you get into your thirties and beyond, says Dr. Dominguez, you can get into real trouble doing some types of stretches. Any stretch where you bend from the waist with the legs straight can be hazardous. Those that require twisting of the spine are even worse. Alternate toe-touching can be a real killer for your back. Also avoid deep-knee bends or squats. A hurdler's stretch with one knee bent and the other straight out in front can aggravate the bent knee. Any stretch with both knees bent behind you can precipitate knee pain. And the ballet stretch with one leg stretched out on a bar can cause hamstring tears if you are very tight. The yoga plow, especially for women, puts a lot of stress on the neck, says Dr. Dominguez.

The real problem, however, may not be with stretching but in the way stretching is done. If you stretch, you should develop the proper mind-set. Tune in to your body and experience how good it feels. When your body is saying it's painful, stop. "The people who hurt themselves keep pushing," says Ron Dushkin, M.D., of the Kripalu Center for Yoga and Health in Lenox, Massachusetts. "Their bodies say 'I'm not ready for it,' and they say, 'Too bad.' "

Introspection

Plato said an unexamined life is not worth living. But others say that at the same time too much analysis leads to paralysis.

There is nothing wrong with introspection on personal problems if it leads to something productive, says Ruth Greenberg, psychologist at the Center for Cognitive Therapy at the University of Pennsylvania, Philadelphia. Problems occur when people think so much that they don't take action. They get so involved in thinking about their feelings that they don't speak to their boss about a raise or tell their wives what is really bothering them or try to negotiate new rules with their children. Those actions would help them feel better, says Greenberg.

Very few people know how to be constructively introspective, she adds. "During productive introspection, you are aware of your own feelings and the thoughts that go along with them, but you're not dragged around by them. You can stand back and say, 'Is it reasonable to think that way or not?' Out of that dialogue can come a very effective and satisfying way of living."

The first step is to identify what you would have to accomplish to feel better. Ask yourself what you are really aiming for and then decide on a reasonable step toward your goal.

When your problems seem overwhelming, just set your mind on doing one thing. Taking a tiny bit at a time gets you moving, says Greenberg.

"If you just stay lost in introspection, just thinking what a mess you are in, there is a definite tendency for some people to stay there," she says.

Physical exercise is one of the most helpful things people can do to get out of the thinking mind into the active body, says Dr. Dushkin. "Just getting outside and walking or doing some aerobic exercise can help them become more in touch with the real world."

Index